Get Back On Your Feet!
What Every Injured and Ill Person Needs to Know

Deborah L. Ribis, RN CNLCP

**Editing by Brette McWhorter Sember**
**Copy Editing by Miriam S. Powell**
**Cover Design by Mark A. Gitto**

Published by
**Women In Print**®
P.O. Box 1527
Williston, VT 05495

WomenInPrint.com
Printed in the United States of America
ISBN: 0-9746109-1-7

---

## Dedication

For my son, Jordan

---

## Acknowledgements

My most heartfelt thanks and deepest appreciation goes to my Jordan. Without your encouragement, inspiration, and help I would still be making notes and procrastinating. You gave my life love and direction.

I would like to thank my wonderful family: Stephanie, Joey, Mom, Michael, Matthew, Ryan and Aunt Mill for your loving support and encouragement. I also offer a prayer of sincere thanks to my late grandmother, Marie Roach; without her love, sacrifice and support my life would be dramatically different.

Thanks to my very dear friends: Nancy and Gil, Monique, Jo, Marybeth, Libby, Clara, Bobbie and Joe. You are the best friends a person could ever hope to have.

Many thanks also to Brigitte Thompson, Brette Sember and everyone who worked with Women In Print® to make this book possible. Your support, dedication and professionalism helped bring my original draft to a completed work. Working with you has been a true pleasure.

Thank you to all the professionals who have touched my life over the years. Thank you to Dr. Gaughan who provided exceptional care and understanding during my recovery. Thank you to Dr. Foerster and Dr. Castine. You are all exceptional examples of what caring professionals should be. You are all extraordinary physicians and I am so proud to have known you in my career. The lessons I learned from watching you practice will stay with me always.

Additional thanks go to the staff at the North Country Center for Independence and the staff at VESID for giving me the chance to regain my independence and carve a new niche for myself. Thanks to Mr. Bishop. You are the ideal of what an attorney should represent.

Finally, thanks to everyone I encountered in my career who taught me what it was to be a compassionate professional; what it was to have strength and determination; and what it was to have such an amazing respect for life and the people in our lives. Every day I learn what a wonderful gift I have been given in this life. And most of all, I am thankful to God for this gift I have been given to share.

## *Reviews*

*F*ighting the system is never easy, even for a veteran state legislator. When you are injured or ill, even routine bureaucratic procedures can be daunting; and if your case is at all different from the norm, the deliberate and inadvertent obstacles in your way can quickly move you from frustrated to literally ruined.

My state legislative office regularly intervenes to assist constituents facing difficulties with the system, including those who are injured or ill, and from my perspective, Deborah Ribis has produced a remarkably useful book.

Her insistence that readers are responsible for their own success, and should not think of ways to scam the system is as important to the patient's success as it is to protecting the public treasury. From the very beginning, the author preaches the critical value of looking ahead, realistically, to making a new life.

Her analogy, "an injury or illness in the body is much like a crack in a fine teacup: you can always repair the cup so it can be used ... but the prior crack remains," puts the problem in perspective from the first chapter.

Then she says, "my injury was one of the best things that has happened to me," forcing her to learn humility along with survival skills, and eventually leading her to a new path in life.

Apart from this valuable mental attitude, Ms. Ribis has compiled a comprehensive and incredibly detailed guidebook intended most of all to give the patient control over every part of the process. At its best, the so-called system is a miserable one, but armed with the information in her book, a person can realistically look forward to getting through it.

Illustrated with many examples from her own experiences and those of others for whom she has advocated, "Get Back On Your Feet!" will make a huge contribution to the well-being of millions.
    *-Assemblyman Chris Ortloff, 114th District, New York State Assembly*

*A* thorough know-your-rights read. This is the type of book that you never think you'll need, but are thankful for if you SHOULD need it. A quick browse through the Table of Contents will convince the prospective reader that everything they need to know to avoid being a "victim of circumstances" is in this book. Ms. Ribis has been on both sides of the issue, and is an R.N. having total command of the issues which she communicates in a fashion everyone can understand and relate to. Don't miss this one.
    *- Joseph Lombardoni, Employment Specialist*

*I* could have used this book when my injury occurred, and I was working inside the system! Deborah Ribis has written a comprehensive, easily understandable layperson's guide to injuries and illnesses. Brava, Ms. Ribis!
    *- Gloria Attar, former paralegal*

*I* found Ms. Ribis' book easy to read. Encouraging healthcare consumers to become educated and empowered is a worthy goal. Consumers demanding more will improve the care received and promote change in the entire system. Ms. Ribis' book provides a starting point for change in healthcare.
  *- Naomi E. Giroux, M.Ed., RN*

*F*inally, a guide to help patients and their families wade through the medical, legal and insurance bureaucracies of this country. This book is an easy to understand, step-by-step resource for successful management. The Glossary of Terms makes medical and legal jargon clear. This is a tool everyone will want to have on their bookshelf for easy reference.
  *- Joanne Gerrish, RN, CPHQ*

*T*his book is written in basic, everyday language all of us can understand.
  *- Monique Lemire, Nurse*

*D*eborah has put all of the medical and legal jargon into layman's terms. This book is invaluable to those ill or injured, giving anyone not familiar with the medical system a way to understand what is expected of him or her and what they should expect from the medical and insurance systems.
  *- Weena Boyle, Proprietor*

*D*eborah is very comprehensive in her perspective regarding cost effective care for the injured and ill person. She has a client-centered perspective, which clearly comes out in her work. This promotes an environment that often drives success and suitable results from medical concerns to vocational-employment concerns. Her level of understanding and expertise of medical case management and effective interplay with vocational rehabilitation counselors have potential to produce great results.
  *- Paul Langevin, MA, CRC-MAC, SDAD*

*D*eborah's insightful, practical, and no-nonsense guide to helping people take charge of their lives after an injury or illness is absolutely indispensable. This book is a must-read for consumers, advocates, educators, policy makers, lawyers, and rehabilitation professionals alike. If you have been injured or have become ill, you owe it to yourself to keep this reference book next to you at all times. I wish Deborah's book was part of my educational curriculum when I was in graduate training to be a vocational rehabilitation counselor. Not only does this guide provide a concise readable and comprehensive overview of our country's system for rehabilitating the injured or ill person, but it offers valuable insight for what rehabilitation consumers must be going through when they become a part of the system.
  *- Jessica Spinelli Sudol, M. Ed., CRC, NCC*

This book is THE book for those who have experienced an injury. It is presented in a unique way by not only relating the actual victim perspective, but also a view from the other (employer/carrier) side. Written by a truly articulate, intelligent, certified, registered nurse life care planner, Ms. Ribis has the first hand stories of life-changing accidents and injuries. She gets down to the grit and shows empathy because of her own personal events as well as witnessing devastation with her clients. This experienced legal nurse offers the reader the education one needs to know in order to pursue the legal issues of working through the system. It is evident that Ms. Ribis has devoted an aspect of herself to being a patient advocate.
- *Libby Turnipseed, RN, MSN, LNCC, CNLCP, MSA-C*

Patients must be willing to take control of their situation and resist passive acceptance. A must-read for everyone.
- *Nancy Zahn, F.N.P.*

I have many health issues and have had to retire on disability. This book would have been a wonderful resource as I was preparing my medical history for the many agencies that were involved in deciding my complete disability.
- *Clara C. LaRose, Retired CEO*

Sooner or later all of us will have to contend with serious illness or injury. We will have to negotiate the maze of medical and insurance procedures and paperwork. There may be legal proceedings as well. Using her personal experience as a starting point, Debbie Ribis has written a comprehensive guide to dealing with medical issues. From the onset of illness or injury to the return to normalcy, all aspects are covered. Debbie writes in a down-to-earth style that is both informative and practical. She does not use technical medical terminology or legalese.
- *Robert E. Cavanaugh, MS. Ed, Plattsburgh State University*

This book is an invaluable tool and is useful before, during and following any illness or injury. For many years as a Crime Victims Advocate, I advised clients to keep careful records and logs of everything remotely connected with their case. I have seen first hand how important those records are and I have often seen the consequences in cases where the patient has not kept careful records along the way. This book is inclusive, straightforward and very easy to read.
- *Gordie Little, Crime Victims Advocate*

Wow! This is an easy-to-read book which is written in everyday layman's language. I wish it had been available when I had surgery. My life would have been less stressful and I would have been in control of my healthcare.
- *Sanda O'Brien, Healthcare Consumer*

*T*his is a how-to manual about navigating the complicated process of dealing with insurance companies, employers, doctors, attorneys and government agencies. Ms. Ribis created a survival guide full of suggestions, advice and step-by-step instructions for getting good medical care, working through insurance claims, getting the most out of a doctor's visit, and much more. With this book, the reader will have his own advocate and guide every step of the way.
- *Barbara Zelinski, Senior Vocational Rehabilitation Counselor*

*M*s. Ribis have given us all of the tools we need to understand the health care system and empower ourselves to take control.
- *Rhonda Mercier, RN, MS, Former Medical Case Manager*

*F*inally!! A well-written, comprehensive guide that is just as important for families as it is for patients. This book is a tremendous resource for ANYONE who is injured or ill. The author's professional and personal experience is evident throughout this book. Thank you for the answers no one told us before!
- *Mary Beth Bergkvist, RN*

## Table of Contents

## *Introduction*

When the average individual sustains a work-related illness or injury, he is left to fend for himself as he wades through the medical, legal and insurance bureaucracies in this country. According to the United States Government Bureau of Labor Statistics there were 1,436,194 injuries which required time away from work in 2002. This staggering number equals approximately 2.7 injuries per minute. And 2002 was a *good* year. According to the Social Security Administration (see www.ssa.gov/dibplan), "a 20 year old worker has a 3-in-10 chance of becoming disabled before reaching retirement age."

As a nurse of 22 years who has worked in the system, survived through the system, and assisted others in the system, it became clear to me that there is not a single comprehensive resource which addresses the issues one faces when an injury occurs, or an illness develops—whether you are at home or at work.

You can review your insurance benefits handbook for your current health insurance plan, search the Internet or call customer service, but none will provide you with the comprehensive information that is included in this book. Each carrier or agency has information regarding their specific coverage, but they don't tell you how to manage your own care. They don't tell you what to do if your care is denied, or even what that can mean. They will tell you that you can appeal the denial and how many days that should take, but they don't tell you *how* to appeal a denial. They don't tell you that their goal is to spend as little as possible on your claim, or that when they say that something is denied or not covered that this might not be the whole truth. The customer service representatives, handbooks or websites will not tell you what to do if you have a problem with your physician or other healthcare provider, your case manager, or the adjustor assigned to your claim. They probably also will not tell you that you should consider contacting an attorney and getting copies of all of your records as soon as possible, or what to do when you do get them. They will not tell you that although you should be able to have complete confidence that the system will do whatever it takes to get you back on your feet, it might not happen without a lot of attention and action on your part.

There are several important steps which must be followed if you are to successfully manage your injury and work towards a successful outcome to your claim. Even if you don't plan on returning to work, you will need to know how to look forward and protect yourself for the future. This book is not intended to help you scam the system. Rather, it is a comprehensive outline that takes you step-by-step through the process. Your initial focus will be to seek the appropriate medical care. Normally this would be considered an obvious first step, but the reality is that there are multitudes of people who do not seek this care or make the claims. Secondly, you must notify the person responsible for the insurance on your claim. Assuming that the injury is work-related, you will notify your employer. Again, this seems simple, but it may not be enough. Once the claim is established, you are then dealing with the insurance bureaucrats and the state representatives at the agency which has the jurisdiction for your claim. All come with their own biases and motivations to move you through the system at the least amount of cost to them. What about the cost to the injured or ill person?

If your injury or illness is not work-related and it will involve taking time from work, you will need to understand how your employer becomes part of the picture. You will need to know how to deal with the adjustors or customer service representatives managing your claim. Your illness might be one that your insurer has identified needs a case manager. You will need to know what having a case manager can mean to your claim, whether you are part of the compensation system or part of a private insurance plan.

Moving through your claim can become a risky adventure. You can be exposed to malpractice which ultimately comes in numerous and—in many cases—hidden forms. You can risk financial and personal ruin while the bureaucrats investigate whether to pay your claim. Professionally, you can be forced to take paths completely different than the one you have been on for the past several years.

An injury can be subtle in onset or come with such devastating force and catastrophe that nothing will ever be the same. Physically, you will not be the same. Emotionally, you will not be the same. You might even have a new job, and you will have found out on whom you can rely and on whom you cannot. You can heal from your injuries or recover from your illness, but you will still have suffered from the problem to some degree. An injury or illness in a body is much like a crack in a fine teacup: You can always repair the cup so it can be used without any obvious problem, but the prior crack remains.

Some of the potential problems can be avoided once you understand the workings of the systems involved with your healthcare. This book is intended to help you, the average person in this country, survive these systems. The medical system which is intended to help can—at its worst—kill you. The insurance industry which should be there to help you with the costs can—at its worst—lead you to financial ruin. The legal industry which is supposed to help can, some of the time; but at what cost? Day after day, you can read articles which talk about the dangers in medicine. You can read articles which bemoan the ever-growing costs of insurance. But you never see anything which tells you, the average, hard-working individual, how to protect yourself. *Finally, here is a guide to help you survive.*

This book does not promise healing miracles, but gives everyone, not just those at work, the ability to take back control of their own situations. It is not intended to replace medical or legal advice. It should not be used to direct your medical care. It is not a binding legal document. It does not provide a promise that every medical claim you have will be judged to be in your favor. But it will, at the least, provide you with the tools you need to successfully manage your claim and your healthcare.

This book is not limited to the workplace injury, motor vehicle insurance, or health insurance arena. It is a comprehensive guide that answers questions such as how and when to seek care, how and when to file a claim, and what to do if the claim is denied or payment is reduced. This book provides you with references that will allow you to educate yourself and arm yourself with enough information to make yourself an informed consumer. You are given tools that can help you manage your claim so that you get the most from your healthcare benefits. You are encouraged to seek legal counsel for issues that affect your medical, financial and vocational outcomes.

I have been through the system. I have seen and heard it all. I have worked as a nurse case manager in the system and I have been a "victim" of the system. When I was the patient in search of an answer and someone to help, I saw every type of physician before I finally found a physician who listened to me and who cared enough, and knew enough, to look beyond the perceived stereotypes. I dealt with the adjustor from hell and fought my own battle with the bureaucrats for my rights as an injured worker. I have worked in the managed care system and I currently work in both the medical and legal systems as a consultant.

My injury was one of the best things that has happened to me. It gave me the experience to be humble. It forced me to survive and find a new path in life. I was forced to give up a career which I loved and upon which my identity was built. I was forced to reinvent myself if I was to survive. I learned to endure. I learned on whom I could depend and on whom I could not.

My new career direction brought me into contact with people who had similar experiences, but who were not fortunate enough to have an advocate to guide them. I hope that by writing this book, I can go on to be an advocate for everyone who is injured and ill in this country. We are such a civilized country, yet we have the most uncivilized, and oftentimes degrading, way of treating some of our injured and ill citizens. I hope that with this book, I can offer the courage for you to advocate for yourself. I hope you find the answers that will help you take back your control. It can be a life-saver to have control over a situation which at times seems hopeless and at every turn tries to beat you down—physically, emotionally, socially and financially.

I believe the true key to survival comes from having a clear understanding of the process. It also comes from being in control. It is most important that you learn to take control of the situation before it takes control of you.

I was a passive patient. I let the situation control and nearly destroy me. The passive patient does not question. The passive patient puts on the patient gown and sits in the cold, nodding and agreeing with the physician or provider, and never finds the words to ask for more. The passive patient accepts whatever is said and, when her condition gets worse, she goes along as though nothing was wrong; again, nodding and agreeing like a bobble-head dog in the back window of the car. The passive patient role is not one which I ever expected to assume, but I did and it was most humbling.

Denial can be a wonderful coping mechanism, but unfortunately it can also be a dangerous path when it impedes your rational ability to listen to your body. A few years ago I fell and sustained a compression fracture in my lower back. As a result of that fall, I was left with chronic pain and problems with my right hip. I was in such agony from the pain, and had trouble walking and doing any activity, but I did not want to tell anyone that I was injured. The plain fact was that I was embarrassed. I did not want my family and friends to worry. I was going to have to change career direction again and give up bedside nursing in the emergency room of a large, regional trauma center. I had finally recovered from a serious neck injury several years earlier, which required a major surgery and left me with ongoing problems from nerve damage and a weakness in my arm. That injury had limited my activities at home and forced me to leave my job as an intensive care nurse. It was a long road to recovery after my neck surgery, but somehow I convinced myself that the fracture nine years later was different. I wanted to just ignore how terrible I was feeling. This is the number one mistake that patients make. It was the biggest mistake I made. I did not listen to what my body was telling me. Instead, I tried to "work through" the pain and ultimately made matters worse.

I am sure as you read this you are asking what gives me the right to speak to you about an injury as horrendous as an amputation, or an injury which left you paralyzed, or an illness which makes you sick every waking moment. How can someone who fell on her butt understand what it's like to be so anxious and sick with worry over money and medicine and insurance and doctors who will not listen and who treat you like a person with a mental illness rather than a physical condition? How can someone with a profession to fall back on know what it's like to lose a job and not know how you are going to meet the monthly bills? How can a nurse know what it's like when there is really no one who understands? How can you compare a pain in the back to a deadly disease? Well, the answer is that no one can really know how another feels, but I can assure you that I have lived through every part of what was, for me, a miserable system.

I consider my injury a journey. On that journey, I went through it all. I am writing this book as a survival guide for anyone who is injured or ill. It is for anyone who needs help dealing with the medicine, the doctors, the tests that don't give answers, the employers, the bureaucracy of the insurers, the state and the legal system. As I said before, this is not a book that will show you how to "scam the system." This is a handbook that I wish I'd had. Instead, trial and error, tears and frustration and pain became my handbook. Experience, despair, frustration, and survival wrote out the chapters. So read my story with the knowledge that I have been where you are (twice), and I am here to tell you that there is a way through it all.

## *Dealing With An Injury Or Illness*

**N**early every household in America is touched by illness or injury at some time. In many instances the illness or injury resolves itself, but it is likely that you will become a statistic. You will have to manage the medical complaints and make decisions about which you may know nothing. You may have to find out what insurance company and system is managing your claim. When you go to the doctor you might not always have the information available to make the most of your appointment. You will need to know what to do and what questions to ask.

According the *National Ambulatory Medical Care Survey*, part of the *National Healthcare Survey* conducted by the Centers for Disease Control, there were approximately 880.5 million visits to physicians' offices and approximately 99.8 million people injured or poisoned in 2001. Even more staggering is the estimated 107.5 million visits to emergency rooms in 2001; of these, 39.4 million were for injury-related complaints. This survey also reported there were over 83.3 million visits to the hospital outpatient rooms in 2002.

### Reducing Costs Impacts Everyone

Every year in this country millions of people suffer work-related illnesses and injuries, and even more suffer illnesses and injuries which are not related to work. Some people even die for the sake of their jobs. Workers' compensation claims cost employers and insurers billions of dollars per year. Employers, insurance companies, and state and federal regulators are continuously working on rules and regulations to limit and reduce these costs. They will be saving money for the industry at the expense of the people in this country. The changes will affect each and every one of us by bringing stricter filing rules and reduced benefits for the average person, especially if the claim is for an injury or illness related to work.

### First Steps

The very first thing that you must do if you are injured or ill is to seek medical care. Do not wait until your workday is over. Do not wait to see if the injury or illness "goes away on its own." Do not wait to complete the paperwork. Do not wait to discuss the problem with your family and friends if it is an emergency. If your injury or illness feels like an emergency, it probably is. For example, if you are at work and you hurt your back after lifting something too heavy, or you have fallen and injured your arm or leg, or sustained an injury from repetitive motion, or you just feel unwell each time you are at work, your number one task is to seek medical care. After you are medically stable, you can notify your employer and file a claim for workers' compensation benefits if applicable. If your illness or injury is not related to your work, the same applies; but rather than notifying your employer you may need to notify your insurance carrier or your managed care company/health maintenance organization (HMO).

Although a hospital will not turn you away if you fail to call your insurance or HMO, it is important for you understand what your insurance company procedures are. Some insurance companies have rules stating that once you are stable, or after a certain number of days or hours, they must be notified. In most cases the hospital will call the insurance company to verify your benefits, but this does not mean you are not required to call also. This applies to accidents or illnesses whether or not they are related to your work. Some insurance companies have rules that clearly state if they are not notified by you or your representative (the hospital is not your representative) within a certain period of time, your benefits may be reduced or denied altogether.

Do not put off medical care for the sake of completing the paperwork. Although this is the rare exception, you may have an employer who gives you a hard time and tries to "talk some sense into you," and suggests that you put off seeing a doctor. There are employers who have belittled an employee for what the employer believes is not an illness or injury worth reporting. The employer may have other employees who have suffered from similar complaints that ended up being nothing. The employer may be trying to avoid additional workers' compensation insurance premium increases by keeping you from going to the emergency room or your physician. You need to hold your ground and do what is best for you.

If you feel you have an emergency medical problem, do not stay at work just to make sure that the day's work is completed before you leave. Do not waste time at home finishing up the chores, hoping the problem will go away. Do not let someone other than a doctor try to tell you what is related to work or not. Do not let someone other than a physician tell you what is or is not an emergency. Many people delay their care because they did what they felt was the "honest" thing. They went to talk to a member of their administrative or human resources staff, they called their insurance company, or—worse yet—they talked to a friend or coworker who had "something similar." They put off seeking care which could have prevented long-term complications. Unless the person with whom you speak has a medical degree and/or training, do not let him talk you out of seeking care or filing an insurance claim—whether or not it is related to your work. If you question whether a certain condition or symptom is related to your work or some other activity you perform, let your physician or representative from the state agency make the final determination.

For example: Jackie injured her shoulder at work. As part of her job, she is required to frequently lift up to 75 pounds to shoulder height. She developed a sharp, burning pain in her right shoulder after an especially hectic day during the Christmas rush. Jackie reported her shoulder pain to her immediate supervisor, expecting that he would begin the paperwork to report the injury to the human resources staff. Instead, her supervisor ridiculed her complaints and said that several other people had tried to make the same type of claim, but they "never got anywhere with it." Jackie was told that if she wanted to keep her job she would keep her mouth shut, and there was nothing wrong with her shoulder (according to her supervisor).

After her weekend off, Jackie returned to work. She noticed the pain was getting worse. She had expected that with a couple of days away, the pain would have gotten better. When she returned to work she went directly to the human resources office to follow up on her earlier complaint to her supervisor about the injury. Much to her surprise, she was told that no report had been filed and they found it "suspicious" that she claimed a shoulder injury after having a few days off. She was accused of trying to get additional time off during the holiday season.

The human resources representative was a nurse. She looked at Jackie's shoulder, told her that she could see nothing wrong with it, and instructed her to go back to work. The pain became so severe that Jackie finally left after just two hours of work. She went to the emergency room and had a doctor examine her shoulder. Jackie was told that she had sustained a serious tear in the muscle in her upper arm. She would need to see an orthopedic surgeon for a surgical repair of the injury. The doctor provided her with a note indicating her diagnosis was and removing her from work immediately. Jackie returned to her employer when she left the emergency room and filled out the necessary papers.

## Listen To Your Body

Any injury or disease can become debilitating if left untreated. Listen to your body. Regardless of who will need to be notified, if this is an emergency, seek medical attention. Once your condition is stabilized, you can make the necessary calls and complete any indicated paperwork. If you have pain or discomfort, call your doctor and have it evaluated or go to the emergency room. If you are injured at work, you will in most instances be covered by the workers' compensation system of the state in which you are working or from which your company is based.

However, there are some special circumstances that can exclude the worker from benefiting from this insurance. There are instances in which the liability lies with another individual, company, or possibly a product manufacturer. This can be clarified by checking with your individual insurance carrier, your state's workers' compensation regulating agency or your attorney.

If it is determined that your illness or injury is not related to your work, you still deserve to seek medical care, whether or not you have any insurance. There are many funds hospitals have available but they might not readily volunteer. You need to ask. By delaying care because you are worried about who will pay the bill, you may actually increase the costs to treat the condition. If money is the issue, seek out the help of a representative from the hospital or your county Social Services department.

**What Is An Emergency?**

An emergency is anything which you think needs immediate evaluation and treatment. Some people are reluctant to visit the emergency room because they do not know if what they are experiencing is really an emergency. In 1986, the federal government passed the EMTALA (Emergency Medical Treatment and Active Labor Act). The federal government's regulating agency, the Centers for Medicare and Medicaid Services (CMS), states that the EMTALA regulations require hospitals with emergency rooms to provide an appropriate medical screening exam when a person comes to the hospital and requests treatment. If an emergency medical condition is detected, the hospital must either stabilize and discharge the individual, or transfer him to another facility that can manage the condition. This law also specifically extends its protection to women who come to the hospital in labor.

Under EMTALA, the definition of "emergency" is broad, and loosely encompasses any situation which a patient feels is "emergent." These regulations are in place to prevent hospitals from "dumping" patients inappropriately to other facilities before they are stabilized. "Dumping" can also occur prior to arrival at the hospital. Prior to EMTALA, there were numerous reports of patients being "dumped" or not screened or treated, or redirected to other facilities because of their insurance status. Several years ago this practice existed as a way for hospitals to limit some of their financial losses when underinsured or uninsured patients presented to the hospital with an emergency. EMTALA regulations ensure that you will not be turned away from a hospital emergency room just because you do not have insurance or money to pay the bill at the time of the visit.

The EMTALA regulations are extensive and carry significant fines for hospitals which violate them. If you are concerned that you have been a victim of an inappropriate discharge, transfer, or redirection to another facility, you are advised to seek the advice of an attorney who specializes in hospital law. You can find a specialist attorney by checking the yellow pages in the phone directory or calling the lawyer referral service sponsored by the American Bar Association in your state.

**Who Has Authority Over My Insurance Claim?**

In most cases, but not all (determined according to the laws of your individual state), the state in which you are working (if this is a work-related injury) has the legal authority over your injury. This means that this state may set the rules on how your workers' compensation or insurance claim will be handled. These rules determine the bureaucratic process that regulates injured workers' care. For example, if you are a journeyman steelworker and you live in New York, but work in New Jersey, and the company that owns the project you are working on is in Pennsylvania, New Jersey's workers' compensation rules *may* have jurisdiction (legal authority) over your claim.

If you do not have a workers' compensation claim, your claim or lawsuit will be governed by the state in which the accident occurred. For example, I worked in Vermont and was injured in Vermont, but lived in New York. Vermont had jurisdiction over my workers' compensation claim. If you have Medicare or Medicaid, the state and federal agencies will direct the management of your claim. If you suffer an illness or injury that is not related to your work, your private insurance, HMO or indemnity health plan will guide the care and management of your claim.

## Different States, Different Laws

Each state writes its own workers' compensation laws and insurance regulations. The federal government felt that it would be a better system to decentralize the industry and let the individual states manage their own injured and ill citizens. There are a few states which do not mandate that all employers provide workers' compensation coverage for their injured workers. In most states, if you have a work-related injury or illness you will become part of a workers' compensation system.

Each state's insurance and workers' compensation laws have different restrictions or regulations regarding follow-up care and treatment. In some states, patients may have the option to see the physician of their choice, while in other states care may be "managed" or directed by a company or individual approved by the workers' compensation system of that state.

## Symptoms You Must *Never* Ignore

It is not always the obvious injury that needs immediate attention. We think of bleeding and broken bones when we are asked to identify the type of injury that requires immediate or urgent physician evaluation and treatment. However, there are other unseen injuries and illness or syndromes that require immediate care by a physician.

### Chest Pain

One of the most important symptoms for which to seek treatment is chest pain. A person who experiences a sudden, sharp pain, pressure or heaviness in the chest and/or arm should seek immediate care. It is possible that strenuous physical work or emotional stressors on the job or at home may have caused a myocardial infarction (heart attack). For *any* injury to the chest—whether it is from blunt trauma such as being struck, or pain associated with non-physical stress—how soon you are treated can determine what will happen to you in the future. Never ignore pain in the chest.

### Head or Neck Injuries

Any injury to the head or neck or sudden, incapacitating pain in these areas should be evaluated as soon as possible. Many times what we assume is just a "bump" to the head can actually cause a serious condition. Our brains are masses of soft tissue encased in the hard, supportive structure of our skulls. There is a cushioning space between the brain and skull which allows for absorption of a shock. However, different types of injuries to the head can produce various types of microscopic changes in the tissues deep in the brain which—if left undiagnosed and untreated—can have a serious impact on your health, now and in the future.

A head injury does not have to leave you unconscious to have a long-lasting effect. There are studies showing something as minor as "heading" a soccer ball at play can cause microscopic shearing injuries in children. A microscopic shearing injury is actually a tearing of the brain cells—causing death to those cells and leading to permanent brain damage in the affected area of the brain.

Sometimes twisting or pulling on our necks and spine can cause long-lasting problems which limit what we can do for the rest of our lives. The slightest flexion-extension (forwards and backwards movements) injury, such as those sustained in very low-speed impact injuries, can have long-lasting, debilitating effects. Injuries that feel like simple strains in our necks and backs can have devastating results if left undiagnosed and untreated. The injury does not need to be immediately severe to send you to the emergency room or your physician.

If you experience a sudden severe headache unlike any in the past, you should seek immediate evaluation.

*Other Conditions*

There are many more problems requiring prompt care than just the obvious chest injury, head trauma, back pain or laceration. Medical conditions such as asthma, migraines, and even some cancers and gastro-intestinal disorders may be directly related to exposures and stressors at work. Air quality and other environmental safety issues in factories are supposed to be monitored by regulations established by OSHA (Occupational Safety and Health Administration). There may be some symptoms and diseases in various body organs which have been directly linked to your worksite or class of industry. It is especially helpful for your claim if you know of other coworkers who have had similar problems and filed claims. If there are others with similar conditions, this may be important information for an attorney should your claim be disputed.

If you sustain an injury outside of work or you experience the sudden onset of medical symptoms after an exposure, there are other agencies that monitor and direct the applicable regulations. For example, if you develop an infection from contaminated water or air, the CDC (Centers for Disease Control and Prevention) or local and/or state Health Departments may intervene. If you are not sure which agency you should contact, you should begin with the local Health Department and then—if you feel they have not been helpful—contact the state Health Department in the state where the problem occurred. If you are still not satisfied and want additional information, you can always contact the CDC or OSHA directly. Just make sure to have all of the information available with you so that your call does not waste anyone's time and the correct information is obtained.

**What About Persistent Symptoms?**

If you have symptoms that have persisted for some time, even though you cannot relate them to a specific date, injury, or exposure, and you suspect they are possibly related to your work or recreation, you should seek medical attention and let a doctor decide if they need to be treated or not. The symptoms may be those seen in repetitive stress injuries caused by performing the same tasks over and over at work. Or the symptoms—for example, those seen in carpal tunnel syndrome—may be related to a recreational activity such as knitting, golf or tennis.

Marie was a young woman who worked on an assembly line putting small pieces of plastic into larger pieces for assembly. She had been doing this job for approximately six months. The orders for the company picked up and Marie began working overtime to make some extra money. She began to notice pain in her wrists along her thumbs from the constant pinching actions. Marie could not identify a specific date as to when the symptoms first appeared, she just knew that she'd had them for a while. Eventually her pain became so severe that she was having trouble combing her hair.

She went to see her family doctor, who referred her to an orthopedic hand surgeon, Dr. Johns. The physician listed the date of her injury as the date that she first reported her symptoms. Dr. Johns gave Marie a slip and advised her to report the injury to her employer as her injury should be covered under workers' compensation. Although there was no specific date of injury noted, the carrier accepted the documentation from Dr. Johns indicating the date of injury as the first date that he examined Marie. Dr. Johns diagnosed Marie with DeQuervain's Syndrome, injected her wrist/thumb area, and removed her from work for six weeks. With the injection and rest, the symptoms improved and Marie was able to return to work. Unfortunately, she returned to the same job, reinjured her hand and eventually needed surgery. Marie ended up with a very small permanent disability of her hands, which limited her activity to anything that was not repetitive. Marie found a new job and was successfully able to manage the small amount of residual pain that she had when she overdid it.

You may have low back pain related to a sacral-iliac dysfunction from too much use of a personal watercraft device or snowmobile during rough conditions. There is great debate that goes on even now between the leaders of industry, the insurance industry and the medical community as to whether these injuries are truly related to work, recreation, or to pre-existing medical "weaknesses" which predispose certain types of individuals to certain afflictions. Regardless of the outcome of this bureaucratic debate, if you are in a position where you are frequently repeating the same task and experiencing pain with those activities, you should seek medical care. Continuing to work through the pain will only lead to further injury. On the other hand, if you have already been resting and treating this type of injury, and avoiding the activities which caused your pain, but you still have pain, it is likely that the pain may be related to something else. You may need further assessment and treatment by your physician or a specialist.

## What About Fraud?

We have heard of people who were diagnosed with certain injuries, were out of work due to those injuries, but continued to have problems that should have improved with the rest away from work. For example, there have been patients with repetitive stress injuries and inflammation who were out of work for over two years, and continued to have persistent pain and inflammation. If they had been following the treatment and rest restrictions prescribed by their physicians, they should have improved. However, it is evident that they either were performing activities which continued to cause the problem, or they were lying about their symptoms and faking their inability to work. They were enjoying the "benefit" of receiving something for nothing. It is this type of person who causes many people to feel that all people who have a work-related injury are scheming and scamming. This type of person causes the insurance companies and employers to be suspicious of all the patients. And it is these people who keep private investigators busy trying to catch the scam artists out there. Many of us have seen the reports on the evening news of people complaining of a work-related injury, such as back pain, who are then videotaped working construction jobs. The news oftentimes reports on people facing criminal charges by the insurance and disability insurance industry for fraudulent claims. Fortunately, these people are the minority; yet they cast a dark cloud on the general population who are honest and have legitimate injuries and claims.

## Determining If An Injury Is Work-Related

When you arrive at your doctor's office or the emergency room you will see that the staff is attuned to people coming in with injuries and illnesses related to their work. Most doctor's offices and hospitals will ask if the problem is work-related, or due to some other accident or cause, as soon as they greet you at the check-in window. It is not sheer coincidence that they ask this question. There are many rules and regulations and forms with which they must comply, depending on the cause of your illness or injury.

Workers' compensation claims are not usually voluntary. You typically cannot choose whether or not the bill will go to the workers' compensation carrier or be covered by your own medical insurance. Usually the laws are very specific about what will or will not be covered by workers' compensation. If your injury occurred while performing the duties of your job, it is most likely that this claim will fall under the workers' compensation system. If your claim is disputed or denied, contact an attorney who can advise you on how to proceed. If a work-related claim is billed to your private health insurance plan, you can be sure that any money which is paid will be retrieved from the workers' compensation carrier. It usually takes more than your own personal desire to keep the employer's insurance out of the mix.

## Keeping Your Ears Open

It is important to be aware of what is said and what goes on around you. Do not discount any information that may be given to you, regardless of where it comes from. The most innocent statement can be the most important. It can be difficult to hear everything, but it is important to be aware nonetheless. It should raise your radar if you hear a provider say something like, "Don't tell me this is another mess from Dr. so and so," or "This is another injury like the one his coworker had last month." Be aware if you know of others who experienced a similar injury or illness not related to your work, such as reports of various cancer clusters in communities throughout the country. Your attention should immediately heighten if you know of others with similar problems. When you hear a statement, or know of other cases, pay attention: It may be more than an exasperated utterance from an overworked physician.

Andrea had worked for over a year and a half in an office that had poor air circulation. She began to suffer from severe respiratory symptoms and went to see her doctor. After a few preliminary screening tests, Andrea was referred to a pulmonologist, Dr. Jones. In his initial intake exam, Dr. Jones began talking to Andrea about when she first noticed her symptoms. He then asked what kind of work she did and where she worked. Dr. Jones, in a very offhanded way, mentioned that he had seen several other people from the same building with similar symptoms. Andrea asked him what she should do. He advised her to stay out of work for a couple of weeks and file a workers' compensation claim with her employer. He also suggested that she contact an attorney. Dr. Jones told her that he had treated several other people who worked in the same building. He said that each of them had needed to hire an attorney to have their claim processed, and then needed court hearings to have their claims accepted as workers' compensation claims. Dr. Jones reassured Andrea that he would do whatever she needed to help her with her claim.

Andrea followed his advice and retained an attorney who was able to use Dr. Jones' information to appeal and win workers' compensation benefits for her. Andrea began talking to her coworkers. As a group they approached the workers' compensation board and were awarded benefits that ensured they would be able to receive treatment and weekly compensation checks to cover their time out of work.

In the months following your illness or injury, some offhanded comment might become the important piece of information which helps you obtain a second opinion, additional care, or treatment which may have been overlooked. If the physician or provider voices concern about numerous problems associated with a certain employer, this should alert you to a problem that goes beyond your situation. It also helps to further cement the claim for workers' compensation, insurance or disability benefits in a claim which, initially, may be denied. If you listen, there is much to be learned. If you hear a statement which makes you believe there are others in your situation, make a note of what was said, with the date and time and who said it. You may never need this information, or it may be a key to successfully arguing for your claim at a future time.

### Keeping Records

When you get ready to go to the doctor, if your visit is not for a life-threatening emergency, take a notebook and draw a basic diagram you can use to show the doctor where your pain or discomfort is. Make a list of the symptoms which you will want to discuss with your doctor (save this and add it to your binder, which is discussed in detail later on in Chapter 4). You can make the diagram and list as long or short as needed. Also, make a quick list of what you have done to try to relieve the problem. It may seem like a pointless exercise, but it will be useful to you later. This will help you make sure that the doctor knows what the problem is and why you are there. It does no good to go to the doctor and then forget to bring up a symptom which may be the most important one the physician needs to diagnose and treat your problem. It will also help you be consistent in what you tell each of your caregivers. This may help reduce the risk of care that is inappropriate or inconsistent with your diagnosis. Make sure to write down what the doctor tells you while you are there. If you have your notes from visit to visit, you will have an easier time remembering if the provider asks you a specific question.

In Chapter 4 you will find a complete set of recommendations which you can begin to put into practice immediately, whether or not you currently have an illness or injury. Keeping meticulous records is the most important task of managing your treatment and getting the most from your healthcare.

### What If You Don't Have Your Records?

Your provider may not have your medical records when you are seeking care. Your medical records are at your primary care physician's office, and if you go to the hospital or a specialist, they may not have your medical records there and won't know your allergies, past procedures or conditions. Some doctors' offices, due to lack of space, actually store the records off-site and need to have them brought over for appointments; so if you go in for urgent care, they may not have the records in the office. Others are moving to a computerized system and the information from recent visits or care may not have been transcribed yet. Or, if it is a computerized system, the system may have crashed or be down for maintenance.

Remember that your treatment and medicines may have changed since your last visit and it is in your best interest to provide information when it is requested. The staff is not asking for the information just to annoy you. They are asking to protect you and to ensure that you have the best care possible. There is legislation that has recently been proposed by the United States Senate which would allow quicker, more efficient access to all of your medical records, but at the time of this writing it has not been passed.

### Be Honest

It is important to be honest with your medical caregiver about the real reason you are there, and about your history. It is imperative that your treating physician knows what medicines you take (including all prescriptions, over-the-counter medicines, and herbal preparations), as well as about alcohol and any other substances used (legal or illegal). Most people are reluctant to divulge this information, but it can cause serious complications and possibly even death if you are not honest with your physician as he begins to prescribe medications and treatments for your individual problem.

### Follow-Up Care

If you have a life-threatening or serious injury, you may have no choice but to seek care immediately. Your claim in the workers' compensation (or health or disability insurance) system begins at that time. Follow-up care will then be planned. If you are admitted to the hospital and you require a surgical procedure followed by an inpatient stay, it is possible that once your condition is stabilized, you may be transferred to a different facility per your particular insurance plan. In many states there are managed care networks which may intervene and direct your follow-up care after you are medically stable.

It is important for you, your family or a friend to notify your insurance if you are admitted to the hospital. In the medical system the term *advocate* is frequently used. Your advocate is someone who is there to look out for your best interests. Your advocate can be a family member, friend, lawyer, clergy member or anyone whom you feel will fight for your rights as a patient. Everyone is urged to have an advocate with them at each appointment and doctor visit. Not only will this help if there is a problem later on and you need to remember certain facts about a specific issue, but an advocate can also make sure that you have your questions answered and understand what your plan of care will be.

Most hospitals do notify the carrier that you have been admitted, but do not assume or expect that they will. The hospitals and insurers usually will be in contact about your ongoing care and plans for transfer, discharge or follow-up care. If you have a problem with a transfer or follow-up care, seek the counsel of an attorney who is familiar with the workers' compensation or insurance regulations in your state.

Once your initial evaluation is complete, and you are medically stable, it is important that you understand the next planned stage of treatment. Make sure that you understand what your diagnosis is, what is involved in any treatment or test, and what the expected outcome will be. Make sure that you have a follow-up appointment as soon as is recommended. Some people will delay their follow-up care in hopes of delaying their return to work or discharge from medical care, as it will terminate their disability benefits. This can backfire. A delay in treatment can actually complicate your medical condition. Some people argue, "The doctor should have known if I didn't show up, and should have called to find out where I was." If you are working with a provider who has only 20 clients, that might possibly happen, but the reality is that most physicians advise you when to return, and it is up to you to make sure that you do so in a timely manner.

The bottom line here is that as the patient you are responsible to show up for your appointments, go to your tests, and get the treatments which are scheduled for you. With the awareness of fraudulent claims becoming more of an issue, you are more likely to raise the suspicion of someone involved with your case if there are large gaps and delays in follow-up care without appropriate documentation of the reasons for the delay.

Catherine had been out of work for months with a work-related injury. Each time she was to return to the doctor for a follow-up exam, she would call and reschedule for a month or two later—or she would not show up at all. She would only call to reschedule her follow-up when the carrier threatened to terminate her weekly checks. Catherine began using any excuse imaginable to delay her follow-up care, expecting that the carrier would continue to send her checks for being out of work. The carrier contacted Catherine's doctor, who recommended that Catherine be referred for an Independent Medical Evaluation (IME) with a doctor the insurance company chose. It is unusual for a doctor to make such a recommendation, but he knew by her actions that Catherine was not working to improve her situation and return to work. Catherine's medical records contained information about her negative work-up and failure to follow up with her prescribed treatments and doctor visits. The IME physician reviewed the information and upon completion of his examination determined that Catherine had reached a Medical End Result (MER), meaning that she had obtained all the benefit she was going to get from her care. The information from Catherine's doctor and the IME physician was forwarded to the carrier and her weekly benefits were terminated immediately.

## Managing The Emergency Room

Going to the emergency room can save your life. The emergency room is often the first medical care that many people get when they are injured or become ill. However, one of the biggest complaints patients have when they go to the emergency room is that everything takes so long. Emergency rooms do not operate on a first-come, first-serve basis. Emergency rooms sort patients in order of medical priority. When a patient arrives in the emergency room with a broken arm, or low back pain, he will not be seen next just because he was the next to arrive. The person who comes to the emergency room with a critical, life-and-death emergency will be the first to be seen regardless of who was there first or who has been waiting the longest. Hospital emergency rooms use a method called triage to determine who is the sickest and who needs to be treated first by doing an initial screen of each person's problems.

When a person arrives in the emergency room, a brief history and assessment of the problem will be completed, usually by a Registered Nurse (RN). The RN usually has had advanced training and is able to make on-the-spot assessments of what is an immediate emergency and what will have to wait to be seen. Hospitals across the country are frequently short on staff, which slows down transfers, admissions and discharges from the emergency rooms. Consequently there are back-ups and delays in care that can last several hours.

Upon arrival in the emergency room, it is very important that the triage staff understands exactly why you are there. There are no quick ways to get around the waiting if your emergency is not considered to be possibly life-threatening. Some hospitals have built fast-track areas which are intended to treat patients who are not acutely ill, but even the fast-tracks are bogged down with large numbers of patients, limited staff and limited hours. The fast-track centers or urgent care centers usually have a specific list of diagnoses and problems that can be treated there. The staff is well aware of what they can and cannot manage. Usually the staff in the emergency room can redirect you to the fast-track after you have been triaged. Most facilities will not let patients transfer themselves to fast-track. The process for transfer from the emergency room to fast-track is also regulated by EMTALA.

If you have an urgent care facility in your town (usually not associated with the hospital), they usually handle what they deem as minor emergencies and routine healthcare screenings. As the services each center offers can vary from city to city, it is nearly impossible to say what specific types of services you can receive there. It is better to research what your local centers offer before you have a crisis.

Having worked in a Level One Trauma Center, I can assure you that the staff is very aware of what emergencies are arriving and at what level of care each person waiting to be seen is. It will do no good to try to cajole, threaten, or be loud and obnoxious in an effort to be seen more quickly. You just might find yourself meeting with the hospital security staff if you become too unruly. If your condition deteriorates, you should let the staff know immediately, and they can reassess your situation. Patients who arrive with chest pains, multiple traumas, childbirth, respiratory problems, active bleeding, etc., will be seen first and usually without any delays. It is always okay to politely inquire about the anticipated wait time, and to check in with the staff to make sure there are no unexpected problems. Do not think that because you have been told the wait is a couple of hours that you can leave and come back in two hours and be seen, or that you can go visit a friend who is in the hospital and be called when it is your turn. If you are sick or injured enough to be in the emergency room, you are advised to wait there. If your name is called and you are nowhere to be found, you will have lost your place.

When you go to the emergency room, you are encouraged to bring along a family member, spouse or advocate. An advocate is a person who will speak on your behalf or at least be there to make sure that you receive the care and benefits to which you are entitled. As long as you make it known to all the staff that you want that one particular person with you, the staff should accommodate you. Your advocate should be able to stay with you as long as she does not interfere with your care. There are some times when she might be asked to step out; for example, when x-rays are taken she must leave the room to prevent unnecessary exposure to radiation. If you go for surgery or have an invasive, sterile procedure performed, your advocate will be asked to step out for your safety.

Regardless of the reason why you go to the hospital, it is important to have all of your information available for the staff. Make sure you know how and when your accident and/or symptoms occurred, and how long they have lasted. Make sure the staff knows what you have tried to do to treat yourself and what has and has not worked. Be honest, and do not embellish. If you try to fib and say your symptoms are worse than they are, this will be revealed in your exam and your credibility will be questioned. When you are discharged from the emergency room, be sure to have a written copy of your discharge instructions, any prescriptions you might need and—if it is after regular hours for your pharmacy—a starter pack of medications to tide you over until you can fill your prescriptions.

## To Summarize

If you are ill or have an injury do not wait; seek the care of a physician or go to the emergency room nearest to you. Once you are medically stable, make the necessary call or visit to your employer to let them know what has happened and what your treatment plans are.

### *Things To Remember*

- Seek medical care as soon as possible for anything you feel needs immediate attention.
- Make the notification calls after you are medically stable.
- If you want to wait, call your doctor for his direction.
- Do not ignore injuries to the head, chest or spine.
- Pay attention to what others are saying around you.
- When you go for treatment, bring a list of your medications.
- Bring an advocate or representative with you.
- Be honest with your providers.
- Follow up in a timely manner when indicated.

## *Questions You Need To Ask*

- Is it really smart, or safe, for me to wait to see the doctor at a later time and date?
- Will waiting cause the problem to worsen and delay my recovery?
- Has anyone else in my community, work or wherever I have been had the same injury or diagnosis? For example, is there a cluster of people with the same or similar problem within my workplace, home, or community?
- Is this something that my employer or another responsible party could have prevented or minimized? For example, were the OSHA or other standards and laws violated?
- Ask the person who made the report and did the investigation to send you a copy for your records.
- When did I first notice the symptoms? What was I doing when I noticed the symptoms?
- Are they getting worse or better? What is causing this change?
- Have I been getting care from someone other than my physician? For example, have I been working with the employee health staff, and is it time for me to see another provider?
- Do I understand what my problem is and what the treatment plan will be?
- Have I started to keep track of my care and organize my personal records?

## 2

## *Notify The Appropriate People*

**N**ot all injuries and illness will be managed by your primary healthcare insurance. As you know from the statistics, work-related injuries and illnesses are increasing. When you have an illness or injury, you will need to know whom to contact and what the process will be. Imagine trying to have workers' compensation or disability benefits started and not knowing whom or when to call to start them. This chapter will guide you through the notification and communication process. It discusses whom to call and how to manage the conversations that you have. It also covers to whom you must *not* talk and where you can find additional information and support.

### Who Is Involved In Your Claim?

It is important that you begin any claim (workers' compensation or health insurance) by identifying all of the parties who may be involved in the claim process. You are the number one person in your claim. Without you there is no claim. You will be referred to by several different titles. You can be known as the *claimant*, the *client*, the *plaintiff*, the *patient* or the *injured worker*. The *claim* can refer to the events and costs of your illness or injury. If you have been injured or become ill, when you request to have certain bills paid, or you place a request for monies to be paid to cover your lost weekly wages, you file paperwork which for simplicity's sake here is called the *claim*. Your *employer* is the person or company for whom you work. The employer or insurance company will be called the *defendant*. The state agency can also be called the *defendant*. If another person—such as another automobile driver—is responsible for your situation, he will be called the *defendant*.

### Who Covers Lost Wages?

When you are injured at work, you will usually be covered under the workers' compensation system. If your illness or injury is not work-related, you may be covered by a short-term or long-term disability policy *if* one is in force prior to your illness or injury. If you are out of work you may receive a portion of your weekly pay in the form of a benefit called a Temporary Total Disability (TTD) check or reimbursement. Obviously, the term *Temporary Total Disability* implies that your situation is temporary and expected to end at some point. If you have an injury or illness that leaves you with permanent impairments or disabilities, or a chronic condition, then you may be termed Permanently Totally or Partially Disabled. In most cases, people who receive Social Security Disability Insurance (SSDI) are permanently disabled.

### Who Is The Carrier?

The insurance company that pays the bills is oftentimes referred to as the *carrier* (for the purposes of this book, the insurance company will be referred to this way). The insurance company is normally a huge organization which is a for-profit business. This is an important distinction for you to remember; the insurance company is not a charity organization formed to support you in your time of need. It is in business to make money like any other business. The insurance company's income is generated with the collection of insurance premiums from its customers. It hopes to remain profitable by taking in more premiums than what is paid out in claims. In order to do this, insurance companies have employees who are charged with the responsibility of managing what is spent or paid out to claimants.

## Who Is The Adjustor?

The person at the carrier who manages your claim is called the *adjustor*. The adjustor has the job of managing the claims that come in for payment. He manages these claims by identifying which charges are appropriate and which are not. Carriers usually have very strict guidelines for adjustors to follow when they adjudicate (adjust the amount of) and pay claims. Although the guidelines are strict about what they do or do not pay, it is important to understand that adjustors keep their jobs by searching for ways to reduce what is paid on claims—or by denying claims altogether. Remember, the adjustor is an employee of the carrier and he is not there to be your friend or trusted advisor. Adjustors have monthly quotas that must be met in order to show that they are doing their jobs. Part of fulfilling those quotas is reviewing claims and identifying which ones can be denied. The adjustor may have limited training in medical terminology, but usually he does not have a medical license or degree. Do not rely on the adjustor to provide you with medical advice. He can direct your covered care, but he may not be able to interpret the results of that care.

## What Is A Fee Schedule?

A fee schedule is an extensive listing of all procedures claimants might receive. If your claim is part of the workers' compensation system, it is likely that the state has established a fee schedule. Disability carriers, HMOs and indemnity health plans—as well as Medicare and Medicaid—have existing contracts which state what fees are to be paid for services and procedures. The fee schedule can be set by a private insurance business, the state or the federal government. In the workers' compensation system, the fee schedule is usually adopted by the state which has jurisdiction over your claim. If your claim is through workers' compensation, your adjustor may adjust the amount paid on your claim according to this fee schedule. By adjusting the amount paid, they usually pay a much lower amount than that which is billed.

## What About Co-Payments?

If you are part of a managed care plan or have a disability plan covering your bills, you should make it a point to know what your co-payment (co-pay) will be. In some cases, the co-pay can be substantial. It is possible that the carrier has set up a fee schedule with the providers who are part of their preferred provider network. It is sometimes possible under both the managed care and disability systems to see a provider outside the established network. However, you need to know that in doing so you may have to pay a large portion of the bill that is not covered under the fee schedule. In some instances a carrier may provide a prior authorization to cover a provider visit or specific treatment protocol. You need to understand additional charges might be incurred which are not part of the fee schedule. Your provider can tell you if they do not accept the fee schedule. In that case, you will need to clarify with the carrier what plan of action you are to take.

You must also understand the various penalties that you might have to pay if you go to see a physician or provider without a referral. You may end up paying the entire bill if you do not follow the referral directions of the carrier in your system.

## Who Has Jurisdiction?

As your claim progresses, you may also deal with a representative from either a state or federal agency which has jurisdiction over your claim. In the workers' compensation system you will deal with a representative from the state agency that governs workers' compensation claims. In the Social Security system, you will deal with a federal employee, as Social Security Disability is a federal program. If you receive Medicaid benefits, you will be dealing with state and possibly county employees who manage the Medicaid program in your region. In the private sector of the insurance world, the insurance company is regulated by the state where the policy is written.

Once you have an established claim, it is very important that you find out who the federal or state regulators are. Which federal or state agency makes the laws by which the carrier must abide? After you determine the regulating agency, you must then know how to reach them. It is always better to be able to take the time to learn this information when you do not have an immediate problem. If you wait until you have a problem or crisis, your thought process might not be as sharp as it normally is, and you might have trouble locating the information you need. Ask your carrier who regulates their business, or do a search on the Internet. If you have a workers' compensation claim, your employer should have the necessary contact information.

### Who Else Is Involved?

In the course of your claim you may also deal with members of the medical and vocational community. A *provider* is a member of the healthcare team who administers care and manages your treatment plan. This can include physicians, therapists and nurses. Most providers will be working directly for you, but some providers are hired by the carriers, or state or federal agencies. Some providers will be utilized to assist the carrier in saving dollars—usually at your expense. They may perform an evaluation to determine if your current treatment is appropriate and meets the rules and regulations per the applicable system.

### The Lawyers

Lawyers may also be involved in your care. Usually you will only have one lawyer; however, some insurance carriers have several lawyers. The terms *attorney* and *lawyer* will be used interchangeably. You can hire a lawyer to protect your interests and make sure that you receive the maximum benefits allowed under the law. The insurance company will hire a lawyer, or team of lawyers, to help reduce the benefits you might receive. This legal team will search for various loopholes and/or develop strategies to negotiate a settlement that is much lower than what you might receive should your claim go before a judge. If you feel your benefits are being compromised this way, you need to find a lawyer to represent you.

Regardless of with whom you speak, or what her title, the most important thing is to know which party in your claim that person represents. Does she work for you or does she work for the insurance company? The answer to that question can mean the success or failure of your claim. It can impact the care you receive. The answer can have significant financial consequences for you, affecting your entire future. See Chapter 5 for more information regarding for whom your doctor works.

### Notification Is Key

When you are injured or develop an illness, it is important to notify your employer as soon as you are medically stable. In most cases, especially if it is a work-related condition, your employer may be aware of the problem. However, it is advisable to notify them *in writing*, whether via your own note or a note from your physician. Be sure to document whom you notified with the date and the time of notification. Document whether this is work-related or not, when the problem first appeared and what you were doing when it started. You will most likely have to complete some additional paperwork regarding your complaint or injury. It is in your best interest to complete this as soon as possible. Be sure to keep copies of *everything*. If you have an emergency and are rushed to the hospital, of course no one expects you to first stop and fill out paperwork. But it is imperative to take care of this as soon as you can. Do not assume that just because your employer knows you left by ambulance that she will complete the paperwork. Most employers will, but there are exceptions. If your advocate or representative is to work with your insurance or employer, you may need to sign a consent providing authorization which allows him to discuss your medical condition and fill out paperwork on your behalf.

## The First Call From The Adjustor

It is not uncommon to receive a telephone call from the adjustor who will be handling your claim. This is usually a good sign; it means the adjustor has been notified or received your paperwork regarding your accident or illness. When you receive a call from the adjustor he will usually tell you he has some questions to ask you about your claim. Many of these calls are recorded. The adjustor will ask your permission to record the conversation. If you agree to have the call recorded, you should tell the adjustor that you agree with the understanding that you or your representative will receive a copy of the transcript of the call. If the adjustor tells you that a transcript will not be made, ask for a copy of the recording. You have a right to a copy of all information pertaining to your claim. If the adjustor tells you that you cannot have a copy, then you might want to suggest he call your attorney and arrange the interview through her office.

The interview call is usually a call to obtain your side of the story about the events that led up to your accident or illness. Remember, the adjustor has probably already talked to your employer if the incident is work-related, or—if someone else is liable—he has already talked to that person. If you are taking medication, it is a good idea to tell the adjustor that you would like it to be on the record that you are taking medicine. You are not sworn in as you would be in a court; however, these statements and calls from the adjustor can come back to haunt you later on in the process. If you do not understand the purpose of the interview or the questions asked, make sure these are clarified for you. If you are not sure of an answer, do not make up something. The adjustor may say it is okay to "guess" or "do your best," but you are better off clearly stating that you do not recall or cannot remember. If you do not feel comfortable answering the questions on your own, politely ask the adjustor to call back when you can have your advocate or family member there to help you and listen in on the call.

## The Benefits Administrator Or Human Resources Representative

Most employers have a designated person, such as the Human Resources (HR) representative or Benefits Administrator, who will handle your claim and paperwork. This person is responsible for the insurance claims of the business. If the company for which you work is very large, there may be different people in the HR department who manage the various forms of insurance the company offers to its employees. You will need to find out whom you must contact. Companies offer many types of insurance, such as workers' compensation for claims (accidents and illnesses) directly related to work, health insurance for everyday illnesses and injuries unrelated to work, and short-term and long-term disability for coverage of time out of work not related to the workplace accident or illness. (In some instances when the workers' compensation claim is settled and/or it exceeds the state's statute on length of time for the benefits to be paid, you may be able to collect on long-term disability insurance if it is available. You will need to check with the individual disability carrier and the state agency regarding the rules and regulations in your state.) If you work for a small business, you may be dealing directly with the owner of the business, as many owners handle all aspects of the business themselves. Your company may also be self-insured or part of a large managed care system.

The HR department will be able to answer questions you have about filing the claim and what happens next. They should be able to tell you if you will begin receiving TTD (Temporary Total Disability) benefits to cover your lost wages and how much that benefit will be. The HR representative will often be the contact person for the insurance company and your employer. Most HR representatives are not healthcare professionals, although some companies do hire nurses to manage some of the claims. If you know the HR representative is not a nurse, be careful when asking for medical advice. You should only be taking direct medical advice and treatment recommendations from your physician. The HR representative may tell you which physicians your plan authorizes, but she should also be able to tell you how to see a physician of your choosing. If she is not providing you with answers to your questions, and the carrier is not helpful, contact the state or federal regulating agency.

## Who Else Needs To Know?

Regardless of who your HR contact person is, it is important for you to develop a relationship with this person so that you are able to have your claims processed in a timely and efficient manner. Not only will your employer need to know about your initial claim, but if you are to be out of work for any length of time, they will also need to have periodic updates on your progress and plans for your return to work. Once you have identified your HR representative, you are advised to clarify the company policy on whom else you will need to update. Many companies let the HR representative manage all of the communications between you and your immediate supervisor. Depending on company policy, you may also need to speak with your direct supervisor periodically so that your time out of work can be covered and your eventual return can be planned.

## Employer And Employee Obligations

When a person is out of work for any time, especially if it is due to a workers' compensation claim, it is not uncommon for an injured worker who was previously dissatisfied with his employer to try to use the excuse of the injury to avoid returning to that job. Employers who are dissatisfied with an employee's performance prior to the injury may try to use the injury (and subsequent time out of work) as an opportunity to terminate the employee or address poor performance issues. Neither situation is unusual. If you feel that you have a problem with your employer, seek legal counsel—especially if you feel that you are being unfairly treated because of your claim. Do not let fear or anger guide your actions after an injury. A lawyer can best advise you on how to handle an employer who is possibly using your unfortunate circumstance as a time to address personnel issues. Most states have specific rules and regulations regarding an employer's responsibility relative to holding a position and what needs to be done to meet their legal obligations regarding your employment. Do not assume that because you have a work-related claim your employer owes you a job.

## Which Forms Must Be Completed?

If you are critically injured or too seriously ill to contact your employer, have someone who has the legal authority to act on your behalf contact them for you. If you do not have a family member who is able or willing to help you out with this, hire a lawyer to manage your affairs. Regardless of who represents you, it is very important to make sure that the proper notification and paperwork is completed. There are specific rules and regulations regarding the amount of time that can pass before you can no longer file a claim, whether the claim is related to your work or not. It may not matter to *whom* you speak, but it can matter *if* and *when* you complete the necessary forms. Every employer identifies the forms by a different name—such as Accident Reporting Form, Incident Report, Event Monitoring Form, or Doctor's First Report of Injury and Assessment. If this is not work-related, you may need to complete a special form to open a disability claim. Regardless of what it is called, just make sure you complete the form and keep a copy for yourself.

If for some reason you have a claim that has not been filed in a timely manner—for example, you develop a condition or have an injury which you thought was not related to your work, but which you later find out *is* due to your work—you should speak with a lawyer about what to do next. It is ideal to have your physician provide supporting documentation when you complete claim forms. If possible, you may have to deliver the forms to the physician's office to have them completed prior to filing. The longer it takes to have the forms completed, the longer it will take to have your benefits started.

## Delays Cause Problems

If you delay the filing of your claim, you may have significant trouble having your claim approved. If you have a physician who will support you, you are encouraged to pursue the claim. If you try to file a claim and your employer or HR representative tells you that you cannot file the claim because it is "too late," call the carrier, state agency or a lawyer to clarify what to do next. Unless you have a signed, written denial from your state's workers' compensation regulating agency, do not rely entirely on the word of the HR representative or carrier. Most employers and carriers are honest and follow the law, but you may unfortunately have the one in a million who will try to deny your claim hoping to save their company some money. In most instances this backfires on the employer and carrier.

## Don't Take "No" For An Answer

If you have an injury or illness which is related to work, but you feel intimidated and do not want to file a claim, you are only harming yourself. It is foolish to try to ignore any medical problem, whether it occurs at work or at home. When you ask someone for advice and they refuse to help you, do not suffer silently and give up on getting the care you need.

José had a repetitive trauma injury (an injury due to performing the same physical activities over and over) to an upper extremity. When he discussed the pain and symptoms with his supervisor, José was advised to "shrug it off," "take it like a man," and return to work. The supervisor told him that others tried to claim for similar problems and were denied. José felt intimidated by the supervisor and returned to work for several more weeks. He eventually ignored the supervisor and went to his doctor, who told him he had a severe tendonitis which had worsened and caused a tear in a muscle. By not seeking prompt care, the pain intensified, the injury became more severe, and an expensive and complex surgical procedure was now required to repair the additional injury. This delay in care resulted in a permanent partial disability. There were many hard feelings between José and his supervisor. When José finally filed the claim, his supervisor denied any knowledge about the problem. The state workers' compensation board investigated and the employer was forced to pay a fine, José was able to pursue care, and he received workers' compensation benefits to cover his medical care and lost wages.

## Employers Value Their Employees' Health

Most employers are supportive and cooperative with the legal and insurance systems. They will assist you with your claim from the beginning to the end. They value the health and well-being of all their employees, and know that a healthy and satisfied employee will work harder and produce more. Most employers understand their workers are human, and humans sometimes get sick or are injured. It is a foolish employer who does not work to bring the employee back and who puts up obstacles for the employee when he needs medical care. Most employers realize that the more cooperative they are, the sooner their employee returns to work, and the more profits they will see.

## The Exception

You need to be aware that there are some employers who are less than honest and will do whatever they can to get around the law in order to save a buck. There are some employers who blatantly disregard the laws. It is only when a person is injured that the problem is discovered. This can be disastrous, especially if the injured worker does not have his own medical insurance. The injured person must begin to pay something on his bills, and often will not have any income if there is no workers' compensation or disability insurance to cover the lost wages. In this case, the injured worker must hire a lawyer who is knowledgeable in workers' compensation litigation.

Martin was working for a contractor installing drain gutters on a newly built house. He fell from the ladder and sustained a fracture to a vertebra in his lower back. He was admitted as an emergency to the hospital and underwent surgical stabilization. Martin was out of work indefinitely. When he returned home after his discharge from the hospital, he called the contractor for whom he had been working. He was told by the contractor's wife that they had not renewed their workers' compensation insurance and that Martin should use his own insurance. The state where Martin worked required that all employers with a certain number of employees on their payroll carry workers' compensation insurance. Martin did not have any health insurance as the premiums were too expensive. His bills mounted. Martin was forced to retain an attorney who filed a claim with the state and sued Martin's employer. Martin's lawsuit took over two years to resolve. The settlement was disappointing. He still suffers from the after-effects of his injury, and has no future opportunity to collect for his bills or lost time.

### Stay On Top Of Your Claim

The state statutes are very clear about the roles of employers and insurance carriers in the workers' compensation, health insurance and disability insurance systems. If you are filing a long-term or short-term disability or a non-work-related medical claim, you will be bound by the contract that your employer has or you have with the insurance company, accordingly. Either way, you will need to stay on top of the claim. Do not assume that someone else, whether it is your HR representative at work or the adjustor at the insurance company, will automatically take care of all that needs to be filed and paid on your behalf. This should happen, but do not assume that it will. It is never safe to make assumptions in this situation. It can be detrimental for your health to assume that anyone will work solely for your benefit. Most of the people with whom you have to deal will be efficient, conscientious, honest, and will follow the rules and regulations established to protect your claim. It is still your responsibility to keep close watch over the process.

### The Uncooperative Adjustor

If you are working with an uncooperative employer or insurance company adjustor, you are urged to contact a lawyer to discuss your rights. Many insurance adjustors are overworked and do not have the time to take care of everything. Some adjustors may be responsible for over 250 claims at a time! If you have trouble speaking directly with the adjustor after two or three attempts, you should request to speak with his supervisor. If this is unsuccessful, then contact the state or federal agency that has jurisdiction over your claim. You can also contact a lawyer. If you decide to contact a lawyer and you enter a business relationship with her, make sure that you understand that her fees come out of any workers' compensation award you might receive. This will be addressed later on in more detail. (Please refer to Chapter 7, Retaining An Attorney.) If you are just too worried about the additional cost of meeting with a lawyer, contact your state's regulating agency. The agency representative should be able to direct you on your next step. This representative may be able to contact the carrier on your behalf to open the lines of communication.

### The Uninsured Employer

There are a handful of states that do not require employers to carry workers' compensation insurance. Some states specify what types of workers are and are not covered by workers' compensation insurance, even if the employer carries the insurance. If you are working for an employer who tells you that they do not carry workers' compensation, and you feel that your injury or illness is related to your work, then you must contact a lawyer to determine a course of action that will best suit your individual needs in the state in which you live. It is the very rare exception where you will work for an employer who is not required to provide workers' compensation coverage, but there are some that simply ignore the rules. Most states require an employer to provide workers' compensation and disability protection for their employees, understanding that an efficient workers' compensation system helps people get timely care, covers lost wages and enables a quicker return to work. Unfortunately, not all employers provide even basic heath care benefits for their employees—let alone workers' compensation or disability insurance— whether it is required by law or not.

### What About The Self-Insured Employer?

If your employer tells you they are self-insured and exempt from certain rules and regulations of the workers' compensation system, you are advised to call your state agency to clarify the issue. Being self-insured does not excuse an employer from following the laws of the state regarding workers' compensation and other insurance systems. If an employer is self-insured, it simply means that they have set aside a sum of money which is to be used to cover any costs incurred under their own policy. They may have another company (called a Third Party Administrator) actually manage the paperwork and distribute the money, but that money is earmarked for the medical costs of their employees. The Third Party Administrator (TPA) will pay the bills from the company's assets and not from a specific workers' compensation carrier. By being self-insured, an employer is making an attempt to cut the costs associated with employee injuries and illnesses. As a self-insured company, some of the "middle man" costs may be eliminated. The company may have more specific reporting guidelines that they have developed; however, they are still required to follow the laws of the state.

## What About Patient Privacy?

An employer who is self-insured for their disability and workers' compensation plans may have their own team who manages claims internally. The same is true for commercial insurance carriers: They have teams who manage the disability and workers' compensation claims. You must understand that when you have a work-related claim, your employer is going to have access to your medical (and possibly your psychological) records that are directly related to your claim. The federal government has instituted some strict regulations regarding the privacy of medical records. These rules are referred to as the HIPAA rules (Health Insurance Portability and Accountability Act). If you have been to the doctor recently, you have signed a HIPAA awareness statement. Physicians, hospitals and ancillary providers (therapists, pharmacies, and medical equipment suppliers) are very aware of the HIPAA regulations. Failure to abide by the HIPAA policies can result in stiff penalties. You may be told that these regulations do not strictly apply to workers' compensation or no-fault automobile liability claims. If you hear from the claims manager that you are not protected under the HIPAA regulations, and you have concern that there has been a breach in patient confidentiality, check with a lawyer; you are always entitled to privacy regarding your health care and medical records.

## What Is Consent?

When you sign your name and give consent for treatment or authorize the release of your medical records, read the entire form before you sign it. Many patients sign their names on general consent forms without reading what they are signing. Many times patients are told that the consent "just allows us to treat you, and then bill your insurance." This may be true. However, the consent may be used for other activities of which you may be unaware. You may not want your information used for some things that are often buried in the middle of consent forms.

Some authorization or consent forms indicate that your personal information will be used for marketing, business and fund-raising solicitations, disaster relief efforts, or used in reviews by various oversight agencies. Although it may be reassuring to know that there is a formal oversight agency reviewing your care, it may not be reassuring to know that your personal information may be sold to a marketing agency. The information may then be resold to various companies such as drug companies and their various partner companies that have nothing to do with healthcare.

When you sign a consent form, be sure you know to whom you are really giving consent. Some people expect and want the physician named on the consent to perform the procedure or surgery. This may not be the case, especially if you are in a large hospital affiliated with a teaching institution, such as a medical college. If you do not wish to be treated by residents and interns you do have a right to say so. If there is something in the consent with which you disagree, cross out that statement and place your initials next to it. Whenever you give consent, make sure you know to what you are consenting.

## Do They Have To Accommodate Special Needs?

It is important that you keep your employer updated on your condition and notify them of your return-to-work plans, as they may still need to cover your time off. They will also need to be involved as you plan your return to work. Your employer can be a valuable asset when you make the plan to transition from your convalescence at home back to work.

If you have maintained a pleasant and professional relationship with your employer, your transition back to work may be easy. Your employer may be willing to provide you with reduced duties and shorter work days, called "transitional duties" or "light-duty" work. If you have been confrontational and not notified your employer regarding your condition, they may not be as accommodating. On the other hand, your employer may not actually have the flexibility to accommodate a lot of special needs which your doctor has prescribed. They may also be bound by certain restrictions imposed by the state regulators. If you have questions, go to the state agency or a lawyer to clarify what your employer must do to accommodate any special needs that you have. There are many misunderstandings about what your employer must and must not do to accommodate your needs. The Americans with Disabilities Act was constructed to protect individuals with disabilities; however, the rules can be ambiguous and may not cover all situations. Do not assume that you are covered by these guidelines until you clarify your position with your lawyer or the appropriate state agency.

## What If You Cannot Return To Your Employer?

If you are nearing the point when it is time for your return to work and you feel that you just cannot return to your employer or previous occupation, you need to notify your employer as soon as possible. It is always better to let them know in a professional and mature manner as soon you make the decision, or as soon as the decision is made for you by your physician. Do not assume that your employer will know that you are not returning by failing to keep them notified of what your future holds. Assuming they have paid the claims, and maybe some lost wages, they are entitled to know as soon as possible if you will be returning to your job. They have a business to run, and the work they do needs to continue whether or not you return. However, you cannot just fail to return without having some discussion with them. Burning bridges this way can come back to haunt you down the road when you least expect it. You never know when you might come across someone in the future with whom you had a poor parting in the past. Unless you move far away, or change your line of work entirely, it is possible that you may run into the person that you would least like to see at your new place of employment.

## An Example Of Poor Conduct

Tony had a falling out with his employer and used his injury as an opportunity to leave his job. Unfortunately, Tony acted in an unprofessional and immature manner, and did not notify his employer of his intentions to quit his job when his doctor released him to return to work. Little did he know that the HR representative he offended at the job he just quit would be transferring to another company. This person transferred to the one company for which Tony most wanted to work. Because of his previous unprofessional conduct, Tony was not hired by the new company where he could have had a better position with improved conditions, pay and benefits.

## So You Hate Your Job

On the other hand, if you are absolutely miserable with your job, and feel that you have no choice but to quit, do not delude yourself and think that you can "make them pay" for whatever you perceive the problem to be. Many people feel that claiming an injury at work, or taking a leave of absence for an illness, is a good way to "get even" with their employer. Nobody wins and both the employer and employee have the chance to suffer more harm. Understand that in some states, filing a false insurance or workers' compensation claim is a felony offense, carrying the risk of prosecution.

## Your Employer Will Be Involved

Whether you like it or not, if this is a work-related claim, your employer will be involved. They ultimately pay your bills. You must keep the lines of communication open. Your path to recovery can be much less aggravating if you are not on an adversarial path with your employer. Your employer can be an excellent advocate and intermediary concerning possible problems with your insurance or workers' compensation carrier. Your employer pays the carrier a hefty premium for this insurance and they have certain expectations regarding the management of claims submitted by their employees. Most employers are honest and supportive of their employees. They understand that if the carrier is not performing in a timely and professional manner, this causes problems for their employee, which can turn an otherwise cooperative and productive employee into one who is evasive, uncooperative and more likely to avoid the return to work as long as possible.

### Inconsistent Lost Wage Payments

This is not does not mean that there are not some employers and carriers who will do everything they can to make your life miserable. There are carriers who will delay or "forget" to cut a workers' compensation check. They may send you part of a week's pay. They may try to avoid dealing with the claim at all, and deny everything. Some carriers inconsistently remit checks, or send them for an inconsistent amount. You may even have to prove that they have calculated your benefits incorrectly. This can be confusing and financially devastating.

Unfortunately, some employers are not interested in correcting these problems as they are self-insured and it benefits them to be paying a smaller temporary total disability benefit. Some employers and carriers expect that there are some people who will not challenge these inconsistencies. They know that many people will not file an appeal when their benefits and claim are denied. If you have a claim denied, or experience inconsistencies in your reimbursements or weekly benefit checks, do not ignore this. The states and regulators have specific rules that need to be followed regarding payments. If it can be proved that the carrier or employer has willfully disobeyed the rules, there are stiff penalties they might face. If you feel that this is happening to you, contact your lawyer or state agency.

### "Their" Interests Versus "Your" Interests

If you find yourself in a situation where you feel the insurance carrier, or your employer, is acting in an unprofessional manner or not following the rules, contact the state regulating agency and a lawyer as soon as possible. Appendix C provides the phone numbers and addresses of most of the states' insurance or workers' compensation regulating agencies. Do not be trapped by an employer or carrier who says that they will "let" you use their lawyer. If they tell you it is sufficient to talk to their lawyer because "he is there to help," do not do it. Their lawyer is *their* lawyer and will be looking out for their interest, not *your* interest. This is a blatant conflict of interest and you should never talk to their lawyer without having your own lawyer present.

### Who Can Help

If you have a lawyer who represents you, you will need to clarify with her how you are to handle all the various forms of communication with everyone involved in your claim. You will need to know how to manage communications with your employer, the insurance carrier and any of their representatives or subcontractors (such as case managers) as well as the medical team. Your lawyer may request that all communication go through her law office. You may be allowed to meet with the case manager or your employer without the lawyer present. Some lawyers want to be present when you meet with anyone, even your doctor. Find a lawyer you can trust, and then follow her advice. You are paying your lawyer because she knows what is best for you, legally. Do what she says.

Some lawyers will advise you to let them get copies of your medical records so they can handle any necessary forwarding of this information. Some lawyers will let you relay the information directly from your providers to your employer and carrier. If you do have a lawyer, it may be best to have her be the point of contact for the carrier as well. Carriers who tend to "play games" with the distribution of workers' compensation or disability checks, and/or delay authorizations for various procedures, are sometimes less likely to be difficult when there is a lawyer involved. Oftentimes the involvement of a lawyer can ensure that delays in treatment are reduced if there are outstanding bills due to carrier neglect. A lawyer can take the problem to the court system responsible for the regulations of the insurance with which you are dealing. This may take extra time, but it may be less time than is involved when you are working on your own with an uncooperative carrier or employer.

## Managing Your Own Claim

You may find that when you initially meet with a lawyer, you are advised that you may be able to manage your claim without retaining legal counsel. Occasionally there may be a unique situation that does not require the expertise and expense of a lawyer. If you are lucky, the lawyer may simply advise you on how best to proceed at that time to protect your interests in the future. This route is not for everyone, and it is in your best interest to seek an initial consultation with a lawyer to discuss your individual situation.

## In Summary

Regardless of who is involved in your claim, regardless of whether the claim is related to your work, the most important step that you can take is to make sure that the claim is filed in a timely manner. Notify your employer as soon as possible to ensure that you do not have lapses in treatment or supplemental income. If you have a claim and your employer fails to complete, or delays processing of, the appropriate claim forms, contact your state agency. Throughout your claim this office may be your best resource. The regulating agency can help make sure that there are no further delays. They can tell you what your average weekly wage compensation should be, and they can clarify the process for approval of your medical care. Finally, they can address your questions regarding return to work issues and special accommodations. The state agency representative might also be able to refer you to a lawyer in your area with whom they have worked in the past to help you with your claim.

## *Things To Remember*

- Know who is involved in your claim.
- Know who your adjustor is and how to reach him.
- Know what your co-pay or deductible is.
- Be sure to notify the appropriate people at work.
- Clarify who needs to be updated with changes and new information.
- Do not use the threat of an illness or injury as a way to get even with your employer.
- Complete and submit the necessary forms on time.
- If you have questions, pursue them until they are clarified.
- Begin your recordkeeping.
- Stay on top of your claim.
- Know to what you are giving consent.
- Filing a false claim is illegal.
- Know what your benefit amount should be.

## *Questions You Need To Ask*

- Who is my insurance carrier?
- Who do I need to call to open a claim? Has my employer already done this for me or should I call? Have all the forms been filed and do I have copies of them? How do I get copies of these forms?
- Who is my adjustor, or who is assigned to manage my claim?
- How do I discuss changes or issues with my claim?

- What is the phone number I can call to get answers at the carrier, my employer and the regulating agency?
- Do I have any co-pays or deductibles? What are they?
- Will I be able to return to my employer or do I want to find another one?
- Who are my providers and how do I reach them?
- How are things going with my providers?
- Do I need another provider? How can this be arranged?
- How can I get a summary of my claim?
- If there is a problem with my claim, how do I get it corrected?
- When I give consent do I understand the answers to the following questions:
  - What am I consenting to?
  - How often does the provider perform this service/procedure/treatment?
  - What are possible complications?
  - What is done to prevent or reduce the risk of the complications?
  - If there are problems, how does the provider manage these?
  - Is this a surgeon who performs a procedure, and then does not want to hear from me if there is a problem?
  - Will the provider deal with the problems or send me to the emergency room or back to the primary care physician?
  - If a new problem occurs, how do I handle it?
  - Are my interests and questions being addressed?
  - Is the procedure the nationally accepted standard of care for my problem?
  - Is the provider more concerned with saving money for the insurance carrier than treating me?

## Medicare, SSDI and Medicaid

Not everyone who has an illness or injury will be covered by workers' compensation, long- or short-term disability, or a traditional health insurance plan. Some people—because of their age, previous disability, or other situation—may be covered by Medicare, SSDI (Social Security Disability Insurance) or Medicaid. Some people who are older than 62 or 65 years of age are on Medicare and have either full- or part-time jobs. Some people have a previous disability—for which they receive SSDI benefits—but are conditionally working. SSDI is a part of the *federal* Medicare health insurance system. Others may receive *state*-sponsored Medicaid benefits, as they do not have enough income to purchase a traditional insurance program for themselves and their family.

### What About Medicare and Medicaid?

For the purposes of this book, SSDI will be included under Medicare. Medicare (including SSDI and SSI, discussed below) and Medicaid will be referred to as Medicare/Medicaid. Medicaid and SSI are jointly funded by the state and federal governments; however, they are governed by either the federal rules or the individual state's rules depending on where the applicant lives.

Not everyone who qualifies for SSDI qualifies for Medicare or Medicaid. There are many people who have permanent disabilities related to an illness or injury who receive SSDI benefits and who have a private health insurance or managed care insurance that covers their medical bills. Some people have a combination of coverage, meaning that they receive either SSDI and/or Medicaid, or they are covered by another commercial insurance plan. SSDI should not be confused with SSI (Social Security Income). Per the Social Security Administration, SSI provides a "monthly income to people who are age 65 or older, or are blind or disabled, and have limited income and financial resources, and who may have never worked." SSDI, on the other hand, is "based on prior work under Social Security." Medicare provides both inpatient and outpatient medical healthcare benefits; however, not everyone has both inpatient and outpatient coverage. The information regarding coverage and general benefits is very complex. Due to the multiple variables regarding Medicare, Medicaid, SSDI and SSI, the reader is advised to call either the Centers for Medicare and Medicaid (CMS at 1-800-MEDICARE) or the Social Security Administration (SSA at 1-800-772-1213) to clarify for which coverage you might qualify. As with traditional insurance questions, if you feel that you are getting the run-around, you could also call an attorney who specializes in this type of law.

### Who Manages Medicare And Medicaid?

Medicare rules and regulations are established by the federal government. Medicaid rules and regulations can be developed by the individual state governments, but there are some jurisdictions which use federal regulations jointly, as well. In an effort to reduce the costs of Medicare and Medicaid, the federal and state governments make provisions for their members to have their care and the services which they receive handled by managed care companies in the local regions. These HMOs (Health Maintenance Organizations) or managed care companies contract with Medicare and Medicaid to provide health care services and manage claims in a way that is expected to reduce the overall costs of the services.

Beneficiaries (patients or claimants) who are part of a managed care network are subject to many of the same restrictions as the non-Medicare members of that same network. However, there may be many services which do not fall under the immediate jurisdiction of the managed care company, but which are subject to federal rules. For example, the prescription and reimbursement of certain types of equipment and medical devices may be different for Medicare/Medicaid recipients than for the other subscribers of the HMO. When in doubt, call CMS for clarification. Because there are still large numbers of individuals in this country who are in remote regions not served by managed care, not everyone on Medicare/Medicaid may be able to participate in a managed care program.

## Managed Care Versus Traditional Medicare Coverage

One very large benefit obtained from membership in a managed care network if you are a Medicare/Medicaid recipient is the more immediate access to care and services from providers directly contracted with your managed care provider. If you have Medicare you will find that nearly all of the providers with whom you interact are aware of the specific coverage limits established by Medicare and their managed care subsidiaries. The expectation is that participation with the local managed care companies will result in smaller co-pays and deductibles for medical services and goods. For those individuals who cannot participate in a managed care program because of where they live, they will be subject to the higher co-pays and deductibles which Medicare has established. Not all providers accept and write off the non-covered co-pays and deductibles established by Medicare and Medicaid. Many will bill the patient for the balance. This may contribute to a financial crisis for the individual under the traditional Medicare coverage, especially if your condition is chronic and subjects you to frequent physician visits and hospitalizations. The rules and regulations established by Medicare and Medicaid are complex. If you have questions, you should contact the CMS office.

## What Rules Apply?

You may benefit from the managed care network with a significant reduction in your co-pays and deductibles. If you have joined a managed care organization as part of your Medicare or Medicaid coverage plan, you may be subject to the same questions and problems faced by individuals covered under disability, indemnity health plans or the workers' compensation systems. You may have an individual adjustor or claims representative who has been assigned to manage your claim, or you may require the services of a Medical Case Manager to coordinate multiple and/or complex medical services. Your care may be redirected or limited to providers directly contracted with the specific managed care plan you have joined. In any case, most of the needs you have—and the benefits you receive—will be based on medical necessity and require supporting documentation.

## What About Problems?

As a Medicare/Medicaid beneficiary, you may find that many of the questions and problems shared by those who have traditional insurance plans, or those who receive workers' compensation or disability benefits, also apply to your situation. When a problem arises you will follow the same remedies outlined in this book for individuals in the other healthcare systems. If you feel that a service was denied inappropriately, you will go to the appropriate agency and follow their appeals process. If you are unable to do this for yourself, you will need an advocate—such as a family member, friend or lawyer—to assist you. If you are denied services under the managed care program which you joined, you may be subject to their rules for appeal. If you feel that there is an issue or problem which is unacceptable, you should contact the CMS to discuss the problem with them if you are unable to obtain satisfaction from your local managed care company representative.

## Prescription Medication Assistance

Medicare recipients now have some prescription medication coverage outlined in legislation passed in 2004. This coverage has limitations. The amount and type of coverage you have may be subject to various stipulations established by the government. Some states have arranged supplemental prescription assistance programs, which help defray some of the costs of prescriptions. These programs are subject to income guidelines and may require an annual fee for benefits administration. For example, New York State has the EPIC (Elderly Pharmaceutical Insurance Coverage) program which assists in reducing some of the costs of medications. You will need to check with your local Office for the Aging or state health department to see if there are any services in your particular state which can help. If you do not have this service available and you are prescribed medications which have exorbitant monthly costs, check with your physician, pharmacist, or even the manufacturer of the drug you need—there may be money available to assist with the purchase of the medication. For example, some manufacturers have established programs for individuals on limited incomes to apply for assistance in paying for and obtaining needed medications. You may have to provide proof of income frequently to show that you qualify for such a benefit.

## Medical Necessity

As with traditional insurance, disability or workers' compensation plans, Medicare and Medicaid beneficiaries will have to meet medical necessity guidelines. This simply means that treatments, services or supplies prescribed will be reviewed to make sure that there is documentation explaining why the service or supply is medically necessary. Admissions to a hospital, skilled nursing facility or rehabilitation facility are regulated by medical necessity rules and regulations. All services may be reviewed. Services may be subject to a denial if certain criteria are not met. If your benefits fall under a managed care organization, you may be subject to additional restrictions. For example, there are some services such as chiropractic care or acupuncture services which have limits on the number of visits allowed per year. If this limit is exceeded, those visits in excess may be denied and the beneficiary may be responsible for the cost of the service. If a beneficiary is in need of inpatient skilled nursing service (such as that offered at a nursing home), the number of days covered and the type of care provided may be subject to coverage limitations established by the federal and state regulators. The type of care provided in the facility will also have to meet specific guidelines which show that the care is skilled and not considered custodial in nature. *Skilled care* is care that must be provided by a registered nurse to meet the specific health needs of the patient. *Custodial care* is care which has been determined to be unskilled. For example, bathing, feeding and grooming are considered to be custodial tasks. Certain types of wound care and assessments would be considered skilled tasks. There are multiple tasks beyond these examples which are deemed by all insurances to be either skilled care or custodial in nature.

## Interchangeable Terms

As you use this book for reference, be aware that much of the material is interchangeable regardless of your particular coverage type. Therefore, if you do not see that the terms Medicare, SSDI or Medicaid are specifically mentioned, it does not mean that the reference does not apply. As with any plans such as the indemnity health plans, managed care programs, workers' compensation or disability plans, you should contact your specific regulating agency to clarify specific coverage questions.

## *Things To Remember*

- Medicare and Social Security Disability Insurance (SSDI) are federal programs.
- Medicaid is a state-regulated program which may have some federal funding.
- Both Medicare and Medicaid beneficiaries may be subject to managed care network participation.
- There are financial and service benefits to participating in a managed care program.

- Not all beneficiaries live in regions that offer managed care participation.
- Many problems experienced by traditional plans can apply to Medicare and Medicaid.
- Medicare and Medicaid offer limited assistance with prescription purchases.
- Medicare and Medicaid beneficiaries are subject to medical necessity criteria.
- Some drug manufactures offer programs which help defray, or even eliminate, the costs of some specific medications.

## *Questions You Need To Ask*

- If I have a disability that is chronic can/should I apply for SSDI or Medicaid?
- If I meet the age requirements, would I be covered under Medicare?
- What Human Service agencies are available in my vicinity? Are there state-funded programs which might help defray some of my medical costs?
- Have I made a list of the people with whom I have spoken, their phone numbers and the agencies which they represent? Do I know how to access their assistance?
- Have I investigated the availability of managed care programs that are contracted with my Medicare or Medicaid?
- If I am part of a managed care network:
  - As a member of the managed care network, what are my responsibilities?
  - What are the restrictions?
  - Do I have to see only their providers, or can I see a provider outside the network?
  - What are my co-pays and deductibles?
  - Do I know how to reach the customer service representative who can answer my questions?

# 4

## *Recordkeeping*

**M**any people go to the doctor but leave before they completely understand for what they are being tested or how they are being treated. It is not uncommon that once a problem is resolved, all information about it is forgotten and/or destroyed or lost. Healthcare is cumulative. This means that what happens to us at one time can affect what happens later on and so on. The majority of people do not ask to receive a copy of their records, nor do they ask to look at them.

When you go to the doctor you are asked to wait in the exam room and your chart is placed in a slot outside, away from your prying eyes. The doctor usually enters with the chart and more often than not, makes his notes in the chart and clutches it tightly as he leaves the room after your care is complete. Have you ever wondered what's in that chart that is so secretly guarded?

Most people will say, "I can't read the writing" and "I don't understand what it says." Many doctors today use transcription services, but some still handwrite their notes. Whatever form your notes are in, be sure you can read them. The chart is *your* history and care. The actual physical paper and file folder belong to the office, but the information is *yours*. If you have a claim for insurance, disability or workers' compensation, what is written in that chart can affect everything about your claim.

### Keeping Meticulous Records

If you have an insurance claim, you must remember that it is imperative you keep meticulous records. This does not mean you should get a large envelope, folder or empty shoe box and start dropping the papers in randomly. Included with this book is a section of reference forms to help you organize your records. You will have more success in managing your claim if you develop an organized file or binder for all of the information regarding your healthcare. You should keep clear, concise records in a binder or document file from this point forward for any care that you receive.

### The Patient Worksheet

One of the first forms from Appendix B which you should complete for your records is the Patient Worksheet. The Patient Worksheet is your comprehensive information reference form. It is a summary of all of your contacts (physicians, lawyers, insurance adjustors, therapists) involved in your care. The Patient Worksheet should be used as your immediate reference form that contains all of your current treatment and past medical history. You will keep all of your records in your binder, but this worksheet will provide you with all of your pertinent information at a glance. It should be the first form in your binder and be updated as any changes are made in your care. If you have a new medication, provider, insurance, etc., make sure you update this form as soon as possible. It is best to update any information you have—on any of the reference forms in this book—as soon as you get the information. You are less likely to forget details if you write everything down while it is fresh in your memory. If you find that your condition and care exceeds the space on the worksheet, add extra pages. Just remember to keep the Patient Worksheet current and keep your binder with you when you go to appointments. Do not leave your binder behind for someone to copy or review.

## List The Providers

Start with a large three- or four-inch ring binder with pocket folders and tabs to create separate sections. You can purchase these supplies inexpensively at your local department store or dollar discount store. Then, complete a summary list of all of the people you contact, including your employer, insurance carrier, physicians, ancillary providers (physical therapist, medical supply company, etc.), attorney, and case managers. It is important that you keep this list current as changes occur. Next, make sure to have a form for each person including name, address and phone number. Also, note if they have a fax number or email address. Do they have an assistant or secretary with whom you speak? If so, note the name. You will add other information to this binder as you work through your care and through this book.

## Separated And Organized

Once you have a folder or section for each doctor, agency or provider with which you have contact, add any papers that you receive from each of these individuals in the appropriate folder. It works best if you enter the papers as you receive them with the most current on the top. It is much easier to access the information if you are organized. *Do not throw **anything** away!* Staple the envelopes to each letter that you receive and make a note on the envelope of the date when you received the document—sometimes the postmark and actual receipt of the letter are weeks apart. Each time you go to an appointment—whether it is with a physician, physical therapist, case manager, attorney, or whomever—bring your binder or file with you. Never give out the original copies of anything. If there is not a copy machine immediately available, let the requestor know that you will get a copy and give it to him the next time you meet. You can also offer to mail it to him. Even if he promises not to lose it, do not give away your originals of anything. They may never be returned to you in spite of the best intentions.

## "We Lost Your Paperwork"

Recordkeeping should be a simple task. It is important to remember that your papers may be the only record you have of the history of your current illness or injury. It is true that each provider, your employer and carrier *should* keep everything, but things can be lost or misplaced. Usually it is a case of human error. It is illegal to destroy or change medical records, and it is very rare that this occurs, but the fact is that it can and does. Most physicians and facilities will keep your medical records for at least seven years after your last treatment. However, if the patient is a minor (usually less than 18 years old; 21 in some states), they will usually keep the medical records until that person reaches adulthood. You are urged to obtain the most current copies of all of your medical records. This should include any lab work, X-rays, scans, tests or whatever is ordered to diagnose or treat your problem. Your physician should have copies, but sometimes files get lost or misplaced. This can be especially important if, later on, you suspect there has been an error in your care. You should be keeping a current copy of *all* of your records, especially if there is the possibility that a mistake was made. I have reviewed records for several years and although it is not common, it is quite possible that another, later copy of a record might be different than the original record you have. It is illegal to change or tamper with a medical record, but occasionally records will be changed or have late entries or addendums added to them which try to explain, excuse or hide medical mistakes.

Most hospitals and larger physician practice groups are moving towards electronic records. This means that your medical records will be stored on a computer, providing easier access and hopefully assuring you safer care. Your physician can quickly reference your most recent diagnoses and treatments. She can see which medications you are taking, if you have any allergies or are receiving any treatments that might complicate your most current condition. If the provider tells you that she does not have a copy of your records, ask the office to please print a copy for you. As with paper records, you may have to pay a fee to have the records printed. Most offices and hospitals will charge a fee, especially if the records to be copied are lengthy. You can check with the insurance regulating agency or your state's medical association to see what the maximum fees are that can be charged to copy medical records. Also—as with paper records—computerized records can be altered. Most facilities have safeguards in place to protect against this type of activity, but nothing is foolproof. If there is the possibility of a lawsuit, it is likely that your attorney will subpoena the office's records logging who accessed your records, when they were accessed and what changes were made, if any. Electronic records have many benefits, and safeguarding information is just one of them. It is not as easy to destroy an electronic document (without detection) as it would be to cut up a paper document and create a new one.

It is possible that the physician or her staff will refuse to give you a copy of your records, stating that this is privileged (confidential) information. If this happens, you can call your attorney, if you are represented by one, and he can obtain them for you. You can also call your carrier, or you can call your insurance regulating agency or state workers' compensation representative if yours is a work-related claim. As was discussed in Chapter 2, there are HIPAA rules in place to protect the confidentiality of your medical records. These rules have been passed to make sure there is no unauthorized use of your personal information. The HIPAA rules allow you to access your medical records as well. As with most other federally-regulated rules and regulations, the HIPAA rules are extensive. To obtain more specific information regarding these rules you should refer to the Centers for Medicare and Medicaid Services website. Although the HIPAA rules limit disclosing personal healthcare information, you do need to understand that if you have a condition that is mandated by your state to be reported to the state health department, or if your condition is related to a crime, your information may be shared with the appropriate agencies.

### Keep Your Records Current

This is your illness or injury. Take the responsibility to keep a copy of your records. If you are reading this and you have been in treatment for some time now, you are advised to get a copy of everything to this date from every person you have seen in conjunction with your care. This includes hospitals, outpatient providers and pharmacies. It may be time-consuming, and some providers may give you a hard time, but you have a right to obtain copies of your records. You may have to pay a fee for the copying, but it will be worth the cost to have control over your records and condition.

### Open Records Act

Most states have specific laws, some called Open Records Act, which regulate how you can access your medical records. Some require that your request be made in writing; others will allow you to make a verbal request. You can find out what your state's laws are by calling your state health department or checking their website. Remember, your search does not need to be complicated. For example, if you live in New York and you want to know if and how you can access your health care records and get copies, do a general search for the *New York State Department of Health Open Records Act*. Or, you might type in *New York Open Records Act*. If you find that the websites are just too complicated to figure out anything, usually a contact phone number is provided that will allow you to speak with a department representative. If you have a case manager (medical or vocational), request a copy of her records as well. If someone tells you that you are not entitled to have a copy of your records, they are either misinformed or lying to you. You may have to request the copy from another source, but you are still entitled to the record. For example, if you have had an independent medical examination, paid for by the carrier, you would have to obtain the report from the carrier, not from the physician who performed the exam.

Insist on getting your records. If you are having trouble obtaining your records, call your state health department or insurance regulating agency and ask if they can provide you with some assistance. If all else fails, contact your attorney and ask him to write a letter on your behalf.

### Read Your Records

Once you get the copies of your records, read them! Do not be a consumer who says, "Oh, I leave that stuff up to my doctor." Do not leave anything up to anybody else. Obtain copies of your records and familiarize yourself with them. If you can't read them, or do not understand them, find someone who can help you. Ask a friend, a nurse or even someone at the local health department, agency for individuals who have disabilities, or outreach center to help you interpret the records. You might be amazed at what you find. For example, if you have had a serious injury and are suffering from chronic pain, you might be shocked to see that your physician is reporting that you are "magnifying your symptoms" or that you are "narcotic seeking," or that you are getting some "secondary gains" from your prolonged disability. All of these statements should cause you to be alarmed and encourage you to either have a very serious discussion with your physician—directly addressing his statements—or prompt you to seek another physician. The records might also reveal a diagnosis which you were unaware had been made, or should have been treated. It is uncommon, but not completely impossible, that you might find information in your records that is not even about you.

If you find information about another patient, bring this to the attention of whoever provided the records to you. HIPPA gives you the right to demand that your records be changed to reflect either a change in diagnosis or a notation stating that you disagree with the diagnosis. HIPAA provides this regulation to ensure that a person's Protected Health Information (PHI) is accurate and complete. This does not mean that you have a right to have your medical records edited to suit your preferences regarding true information which you rather not have documented for some reason. A medical record is a legal document. If there is something in it with which you disagree, or know to be inaccurate, send a letter to your doctor explaining that your letter is to be included with your records. Be specific in your letter when detailing what you feel is inaccurate and why it needs to be changed. Make sure to keep a copy of any such correspondence for your own records. If possible, send the letter with a return-receipt requested to verify that it was received. This does not apply just to your doctors. It can apply to your hospital records, physical therapists and case managers, or whoever is involved in your claim.

## Extra Binders Needed

As you start to acquire your records, you may find that you need a second or even a third binder if your treatment has been going on for a long time. For one year of treatment, you may have a file drawer which is nearly full. If you cannot keep your own records, find a friend, family member or attorney who can help. Again, do not get rid of anything, and do not assume that the carrier or your employer or physician will have everything that you might need. They might have it, but they might not cooperate in sharing it with you.

As you begin to request your records, you should be asking for copies of those records in their entirety. The carrier has a medical file, but they also have claims notes or internal communication logs. Your attorney might need to get these with a subpoena, but they can explain a lot, especially if you are running into obstacles with your care. Physicians are sometimes reluctant to hand over the records. Make it clear that you want their entire record, including all of their handwritten and dictated information. There may be a huge difference in the scribbled notes from the few minutes you spend in the office and the dictated notes which refer to the visit.

## Log Your Contacts

Always keep a log which includes the name of the people to whom you talk, when you talk to them and any notes about the conversation. For example: "02-11-99 at 2:30 p.m., notified *Sue* at work that I saw Dr. Bob and he wants me to go to physical therapy." Keep your log in order; it will save you a tremendous amount of aggravation and time if you have to look something up later. Keep your contact log in a separate tabbed section in your binder. Your contact log will become a diary of sorts. It will be your memory of what happened, when it happened, and who was notified. This can be very valuable, especially if the claim is challenged. Do not assume that anyone but you will keep records of what was done. If you are later challenged about a phone contact, there will usually be documentation either on your phone bill (showing you placed the call) or on the phone bill of the person who called you. If your home or cellular phone bill arrives and has proof of relevant calls on it, add it to the contact log section of your binder.

## Make A Note

Regardless of how insignificant you think the visit, call or written information is, make sure to make an entry in your contact log or diary about every contact. No matter how good your memory, you may not be able to remember every single detail a few days, months or years afterwards. When people are under stress they have a hard time remembering specific details. At the start of your recordkeeping, you should write a summary of anything that you can remember about your symptoms or injury. It may be easiest at first to just jot down random statements, and then afterwards try to put them into a paragraph or even a simple timeline. Use whatever form you find most comfortable, but do this as soon as you can. If you are taken to the hospital, have a family member, friend or attorney start to keep these notes for you. You will be asked multiple times over the course of your illness or injury—and throughout your claim—to review what has happened thus far. It will be much easier to be consistent if you have a written summary to which you can refer.

## The First Report

Another important form which you will want to have, if your injury is work-related, is a copy of your Incident Report, Accident Report, First Report of Injury, or whatever the notification form that your company uses to report your illness or injury. Make sure to get a copy of this from your employer, or—if you have not completed one yet—make a copy for yourself before you hand it in. Once it has been completed by your employer to initiate a workers' compensation claim, obtaining a copy of the First Report of Injury is very important. There may have been additions of which you are not aware. If a disability claim or insurance claim form is completed, keep a copy for your records. Whenever you receive a letter or form that you need to "sign and return," you must keep a copy of this as well—even if they promise to send you back a copy. If you send anyone anything, *always keep a copy!* By keeping a copy of your documentation with the dates on it, you can prove that you met your obligations under the requirements of the state or insurance.

## Make Sure It Can Be Traced

If you have to have forms signed and returned to a state agency, the carrier, or an employer, and they are to be returned by a specific date, you should return these forms by some form of traceable mail carrier. The U.S. Postal Service and all of the commercial postal/parcel carriers have various delivery methods to trace and guarantee that your letter or package arrives at a specific time and place by a specific date. This can be important, especially if there is the possibility that you may be up against a deadline for filing your claim. If you are worried about meeting a deadline, contact an attorney for his assistance in either obtaining an extension or making sure that the report is filed on time. When you send a letter to the carrier or state agency, you may need the postal tracking record to prove when you sent out the package and when it was received. This will be especially helpful if you are told that it was never received. With a record of your transaction, and a signature of receipt from the company that you addressed, you will have proof that they did receive your letter and it was not lost in the mail.

Proving what you sent and when you sent it can be especially important when it comes time to file an appeal—especially if the contract limits your time to appeal a decision. Be sure to keep a copy of anything you send out and add it to your binder under the appropriate heading. Also, make a notation of all such correspondence in your log to keep the contact information up-to-date. Keep copies of mailing receipts showing how much you paid the Post Office or commercial mailing service. If your carrier requires that information is sent via special handling, such as return-receipt requested, or by certified mail (which costs additional postage and delivery fees), keep this receipt and submit it for reimbursement from the carrier.

## Print The Email

If you communicate with anyone by email, make sure to print out copies of everything that you send and receive and add them to your binder. Also, save copies of any communication on a disc or your computer hard drive to make certain that the communication is preserved.

## Travel And Appointment Logs

After you begin your communication log, you should also start a Travel/Mileage and Appointment log. Many states will reimburse for mileage to and from various appointments associated with workers' compensation claims. Each state has very specific rules and regulations regarding reimbursement; you will need to check with your local agency. Do not rely on information about travel reimbursement from your employer, doctor or friends. Your state agency can explain the specific requirements. For example, some will only reimburse you for mileage that is more than what you would travel to work each day. Unfortunately, not all states provide reimbursement. To find out if your state reimburses for mileage for a workers' compensation claim, contact the workers' compensation regulating agency in your state.

Once you know what your state covers, check with the carrier to find out how often they want you to submit your mileage reimbursement request. If/when you do submit a mileage reimbursement request, make sure to keep the original copy. If your carrier requires original receipts for ferry or toll fees, be sure to keep a copy for your file. These are frequently lost or never received by the carriers and need to be resubmitted. It might not seem worth the trouble to keep track of your mileage, but if—for example—the reimbursement rate is thirty-nine cents a mile and you travel forty miles three times a week for physical therapy, you could be looking at a reimbursement of about $46.80 a week. Again, not all state's workers' compensation coverage allows for mileage reimbursement, but it is worth investigating. If you have a liability claim, you might discuss mileage and travel costs with your lawyer to see if you should be keeping receipts and accurate mileage records for your future claims settlement discussions.

## Bring A List Of Questions

Now that you understand that you must keep a copy of everything and make a note of everyone with whom you communicate, you need to make a list of written questions and issues to discuss at your next doctor's appointment. If the doctor cannot, or will not, take the time to help you fill out the form with written answers, you should take a few minutes to write down what the doctor told you before you leave the office or parking lot. The longer that your postpone making your notes, the more likely you are to forget some important points. When you leave your doctor's office, you will most likely have a form (sometimes it's just a scribbled note on a prescription pad) about your work status, treatment plan or prescription medication, as well as an appointment for follow-up with the physician. If you ask, most office assistants will make a copy of all of this for you. Make sure to get any forms copied before you distribute them. When you get home, add your copies to your binder under the appropriate heading.

If you are still confused about what the doctor said, do not leave his office without getting the information you need. Ask a nurse or staff member to help you, but do not leave with unanswered questions.

## Keep Your Reference Materials

As you progress with treatment, you may also receive various articles or pamphlets related to your illness or injury. You may even receive an informational packet from the insurance or workers' compensation system handling your claim. Make a separate tab in your binder and keep these materials for later reference. If you are reading a magazine or newspaper and see an article which you think pertains to your situation, cut it out or make a copy for your binder. If you hear something mentioned on the news that you think might help, try to contact the radio or television station, or check their website for the information. Always try to get something in writing for your reference section of your binder. The next time you meet with your physician, and you have your binder, you will have the reference information ready to discuss with him.

## The Investigator's Report

You are also entitled to a copy of any investigator reports. Due to the increased number of fraudulent claims, many carriers contract with private or field investigators. These are investigators who will approach you directly, or follow you and film you for a certain period of time. If you suspect that you have been followed and taped, contact an attorney. Obtain a copy of the tape and the written report. Many state regulating agencies may view the tape or surveillance as inadmissible if your case goes to court.

If there is a tape that shows you doing something without the usual difficulties you have had since your illness or injury began, the report might impact the direction the carrier goes with your claim. The carrier may not believe that you are having the trouble and limits you say you do and may decide to deny your claim, or send you to their physician for an independent medical exam to have your claim closed. If this happens and you go to court to appeal the action the carrier takes, it is helpful for you to have the investigator's report and any tape that was made. You may be able to convince the court you were having a good day and were able to do more than you can do most other days.

If you are having a better-than-average day, and are able to increase your activity, you should make a note of this in your log and discuss it with your physician at your next appointment. It may help you later if your claim is challenged by the witness account of your activity, especially if you can produce a diary which indicates what was happening on the day in question. Some patients who have extreme fluctuations from day to day get a calendar and make a plus or minus sign on each day if keeping a diary is too much of a chore.

If you are working and it is proved (on videotape) that you are able to work, you may be faced with immediate termination of your benefits and charged with insurance fraud.

## The Reimbursement Record

The forms in Appendix B provide a Reimbursement Record. You will probably want to make additional copies of this form, especially if your claim is going to take a long time to resolve. You will want to use this to keep track of any money you pay out in connection with your care. For example, if you make a co-pay for a service or pay out-of-pocket for your medications, make sure to note it on the Reimbursement Record. If you submit a copy of the receipt, make sure to retain your own copy as well, and make a note of when you submitted it to the carrier. Once you receive reimbursement for the money you paid, make a note of the reimbursement on your record.

You may want to begin your Reimbursement Record by attaching a copy of your last three to four months' paychecks. If you are a workers' compensation recipient, many states compute how much compensation you receive based on your average weekly wage (AWW). You should find out how many weeks your state uses and gather up all of your pay stubs. You will receive a letter from the workers' compensation division which will explain what your compensation will be. Keep this letter with your Reimbursement Record. More importantly, review all of your pay stubs to verify that there are no discrepancies. If the carrier overpays you, you could have to pay it back. If you are underpaid, you will want to have a way to dispute the difference. This is an excellent place to keep a log of any checks—such as disability or workers' compensation—which you receive.

Most people will argue that this is just extra work, but if you are having trouble getting your checks, or they are consistently a day or two late, over time—if you count up the delays—you might find that you are missing a week's or even a couple of weeks' disability or compensation. Most disability or compensation checks have a stub attached to them. It is a good idea to attach these stubs to the reimbursement record to keep an orderly summary of your money.

## The Appointment Log

The Appointment Log is included in Appendix B to help you keep track of your appointments. If you have your binder with you at each appointment, you can use the Appointment Log to make a note about when your next appointment is. This is especially helpful if you do not keep accurate notes on a calendar. The Appointment Log can also provide you with a summary of your care if there is a question in the future about which appointments you kept and which appointments you might have missed.

## In Summary

It is imperative that you have one place to put everything related to this illness or injury. Even if you do not want to keep an organized binder, make sure you keep all of your records together. Do not mix up these papers with your other household papers or—worse yet—throw them out. They may be the only record that you will have if there is any need to argue for your claim. Once your claim is settled, continue to keep these records in a safe place. You may need them in the future if you have a recurrence of all or part of your condition. They will be a helpful tool later on if you need to provide a summary of past medical or surgical care. If you use your binder correctly and keep the information current, it can help you maintain control over your care, and it can help you dispute any future questions about your entire claim. There can be a lot of information to enter and track, but if you have an injury or illness and are not able to work, you should be able to find the time to keep your information updated. If you are unable to do it for yourself, ask a family member or friend to help you.

### *Things To Remember*

- Keep meticulous records.
- Make a list of your contacts.
- Keep different information in separate folders.
- Do not throw anything away.
- Keep your records current.
- Read your records.
- Write a summary of events.
- Get a copy of all reports.
- Make sure to send mail that can be traced.
- Print and save your emails.
- Keep Mileage/Travel, Appointment and Contact logs.
- Bring a list of questions with you to each doctor appointment.
- Bring your binder or file with you to appointments.
- Write down what has been told to you.
- Keep any reference information you are given.
- Get the investigator's report.
- Remember, a written record is better than your memory.

### *Questions You Need To Ask*

- What is the name, phone number, address and fax number for each of my providers?
- Do I have all of the information that I need to complete my Patient Worksheet?
- Have I set up an organized filing system, in chronological order, so I have everything at my fingertips?
- Have I obtained current (and past) copies of my entire record—including the claims history—from all involved in my claim?

- If I am sending a report or bills for reimbursement, have I kept a copy for my records?
- Do I have copies of the tracking receipts for any correspondence I sent?
- Have I backed up my email used to communicate with those involved in my claim?
- If I am dealing with the insurance carrier, have I requested a copy of their records, as well as their interoffice communication log or claims notes? If not, has my attorney?
- Have I completed my Reimbursement Record and attached copies of any receipts that I have paid?
- Have I kept an accurate record of my disability or workers' compensation checks?
- Are my payments timely and accurate, or is there a pattern of delays showing that the carrier owes me for a week or more of missed payments?

# 5

## *Educate Yourself: Take Control*

Part of surviving any illness or injury is being able to understand what is happening to you and why it is happening. Ignorance about your condition only adds to the stress. You are already vulnerable because of the illness or injury. Not understanding what is happening, and leaving everything about your care and your claim to the others involved in the claim, places you in a compromised position. When you do not have all the facts, you give up control of what happens to you.

### Do Not Assume Anyone Knows Everything

One of the most important things you can do is to *educate yourself* about your illness or injury. To assume that your caregivers (doctors, nurses, therapists, etc.) will always make the best decisions is risky. Your providers may be highly-educated professionals with advanced and specialized training, making decisions guided by their training, experiences and understanding of traditional treatment protocols. There are always new discoveries and treatment alternatives being developed.

However, there is not a person alive who knows all there is regarding a specific illness or injury. Do not assume that your providers know everything and—most of all—do not assume that their plans and motives are solely for your best interest. Most physicians are honest and forthcoming with their patients. Some are not. As with any group of people, there are some who have their own agendas and find it difficult to objectively manage certain situations without inflicting their own biases. If your physician tells you he has the only answers available, and that he knows everything there is about your condition, you are urged to find a new doctor as soon as possible. Only a very egotistical person presumes to know everything. You need someone who is open to you and your needs, not someone who has preconceived ideas.

### Know Your Options

If you do not understand what your options are, you cannot make an informed choice. Many physicians will make a plan, only to have it changed when a patient either presses for more answers or presents alternate treatment options. This does not mean that every new therapy or treatment you read about will be appropriate for your situation. But if you are unaware of your options, you will never know what the chances for an alternate solution to your problem might be. For example, if you are told that the only way to treat a certain injury is with time, and then two years later you find out that the delay caused more problems, your situation will be worse. If your doctor is unwilling to discuss possible options, ask for a referral to another caregiver with whom you can explore other available possibilities.

### The Doctor's Mind May Be Closed

Some physicians may close their minds to any other treatment considerations or diagnostic possibilities. It is usually obvious that these physicians may be unconcerned and unwilling to pursue anything other than their "standard" treatment options. If you are not improving with the current treatment plan—or are getting worse instead of better—and your physician will not listen to your questions or complaints, you *must* find another physician. Do not let his agenda stand in the way of your recovery. If the physician tells you that he "won't be told what to do," you should consider ending the relationship immediately. Remember, medicine is a business and you are a customer. If you are not satisfied, you need not make the purchase.

You can call your local health agencies or community support groups (such as your local chapter of the Fibromyalgia Support Network, for example) for help; they are there to offer support and resources to people in the community with various diagnoses. These agencies and groups can help you find another physician who may be better suited to your particular situation. You will need to do research and learn about your diagnosis. Learning about your condition and asking questions will help you find a specialist who understands your diagnosis. Once you find a doctor who is truly interested in helping you manage and/or overcome your illness or injury, you will be able to start healing and reclaim control of your situation. Providing new information to your provider or asking for an alternative treatment should not feel uncomfortable or threatening. It is unprofessional for a doctor to ignore or walk away from a patient who still has questions. If your doctor answers your question by telling you he "doesn't know" the answer, then you need to ask him to refer you to someone who might know. It is always preferable to respect someone admitting he does not know the answer, than to suffer silently while someone pretends he knows everything.

## Make Sure The Report Is Accurate

Your troubles may not end when you find a new physician. It is rare, but there are physicians who become angry if you ask for a referral to another doctor for another opinion. It is your right as a patient to seek care from whomever you choose. You have a right to seek out another opinion without worrying about the feelings of the doctor treating you.

If you fear your doctor might retaliate by discharging you from his care, or if you worry he might pass on a false report to the carrier, obtain copies of your records immediately (before you leave the office). Although it is not common, there are some physicians who will pass a report to the carrier which is either inaccurate or embellished. They do this in hopes that the carrier will deny your transfer to another provider. Once you have your reports, review them immediately for inaccuracies and offending language. If the report is incorrect in any way, you will have to write a letter to the doctor who made the report, asking him to correct the error. This letter should be copied and sent to the state representative overseeing your case, and to the adjustor managing your claim.

If you are dealing with your private insurance, it is possible that your insurance company requires your medical records accompany the bills. Payment or denial of these bills may be determined by what is written in those records. If you find that there are inaccuracies in your medical records, you should send a letter to whomever wrote the report and provide a very specific reason why you feel the information is wrong. Explain what you think would be an accurate statement or report. If you find out that the faulty report was sent along with the bill to your insurance company, you should copy them on your letter. If the doctor will not provide what you believe to be an accurate report of your assessment, you can discuss this with a call and follow-up letter to the local medical association. If you have been denied benefits based on an inaccurate statement by a physician, and the physician will not amend his report to reflect this error, then you may need to retain an attorney to help fight for your benefits.

Unfortunately, it may be up to you to prove that the report is false and inaccurate. This may be where your explicit recordkeeping can clear up any misinformation and untrue statements that may be circulating about you. Without your accurate files you might not be able to disprove these statements. This is very important because the false report may be used by the carrier as an opportunity to terminate your benefits. This can have devastating physical, emotional and financial results.

You must always remember that the adjustor is looking for the opportunity to reduce the amount of money spent on your claim. This is how insurance companies stay in business. They keep their profits up by limiting what they pay out. If your claim is denied, it will be up to you (or your lawyer) to file an appeal. This is especially important if you feel that you need more care, which is now financially unavailable because your claim has been closed. If you hope to successfully have the denial overturned, you may have to do some more research. You may need to provide a written appeal supported by all of the information in your file, along with any documentation you may have from your new physician. The appeals process can be very challenging and intimidating. If you have any questions at all, you should hire an attorney to help you with the appeal. The amount you have to pay a lawyer may be worth every penny to help get your benefits reinstated.

## For Whom Does Your Doctor Work?

You must educate yourself about who your doctor or provider is. You must find out for whom they work and with whom they contract. If your employer has hired or contracted with the doctor you are seeing, it is possible that the doctor will be less than aggressive in his diagnosis and treatment of your problem. Some doctors who operate occupational medicine or physical medicine and rehabilitation practices have contracts with many employers in their regions. Some of these physicians and providers have unspoken and unwritten agreements with these employers. They will care for and treat the employers' injured workers, but with the goal of returning the injured workers back to their jobs as soon as possible, while spending minimal money on diagnostics, treatment and referrals. If you are referred to a physician who is employed by your company—or who has a contract with your employer—you should consider getting another opinion from a physician unaffiliated with your workplace.

A conflict of interest arises when one group (the doctors) works for another group (the employers) and is also supposed to provide service (healthcare treatment) for a third group of people (the injured workers). This conflict of interest can often work against the injured worker, with the only benefit being to the employer who holds the contract with the physicians. The employer benefits because the costs to diagnose and treat the injured worker are kept to a minimum and there are frequently no lost wages paid out because the injured worker is not excused from work. This helps keep the employer's workers' compensation premiums at a lower rate. Each time there is a claim, especially if it is an expensive claim, the workers' compensation insurance premiums increase. The physician benefits by getting more referrals from the employers. In a situation such as this, you should see your own physician even if it means paying out-of-pocket. The same can be said if you have a non-work-related illness and receive disability benefits through your employer's plan. If you request another opinion and the physician or your employer denies your request, you can usually appeal to your state agency for authorization to change providers—especially if you can prove that there is a relationship between your employer and the doctor they sent you to see.

These physicians earn their living and benefit from their referral relationship with your employer. Their reports and evaluations about your illness or injury may not always reflect the seriousness of your injury or claim. If you read their reports, you might find that they have left out key parts of your injury or illness. The reports might not mention the biggest complaints or discomforts that you bring to the doctor and his staff. The physician's relationship with your employer may be much stronger than the relationship you have with the doctor. When this is the case, your doctor's interest is best served by providing information which hastens a closure or denial of your claim. By saving money for your employer, he proves his worth to them, and continues to receive their referrals. Successful work for one employer may generate additional work with other employers. This may be especially evident for workers' compensation beneficiaries or members of group health plans that are employer-financed (self-insured). Many physicians or groups who market occupational medicine services provide documented evidence of the savings they have provided for other employers. If this were untrue, companies specializing in occupational medicine would not provide employers with reports like cost/savings analyses.

## The Physician Specialist

Once you know who your physician or provider is, and for whom he works, do some more research to determine in what area of medicine he specializes and what his certifications are. You can usually find this information at the American Medical Association website's Doctor Finder page (www.ama-assn.org). It is important to know your physician's specialty. You can also check the American Board of Medical Specialties (www.abms.org) to verify your physician's specialty certification. Each specialty in medicine is governed by a set of standards specific to that discipline. For example, the orthopedic surgeon follows certain standards which guide him when managing low back pain. Those standards and treatment options may be very different than how a physical medicine and rehabilitation specialist (physiatrist) would treat the same problem.

It is uncommon for a physician not to be affiliated with a professional organization in his specialty. Do some research about your diagnosis and find out what specialist is most appropriate to treat your problem. If you want some general information about what type of professional manages low back pain, for example, just do a search with a question like "who treats low back pain?" The responses will be staggering. You will see that back pain can be managed by multiple types of physicians, all of whom have very different goals and objectives when they treat.

If you have chronic pain, for example, you may want to be evaluated by a physician who specializes in chronic pain syndrome. You might consider a referral to a pain management specialist. You might see a neurologist, an anesthesiologist or a rehabilitation specialist. Not all physicians specialize in management of chronic pain. All doctors have training, theories and experience used to manage pain, but pain management can be its own specialty. If you have an orthopedic problem, it may not be in your best interests to see a general practitioner exclusively. For example, if you have a repetitive stress injury in the wrist, you may want to see an orthopedic or hand surgeon who specializes in diseases and conditions of the upper extremities, as opposed to a general orthopedist. The general orthopedist may know all there is to know about bones and joints throughout the body, but there may be more specialized treatment options for the wrist which might improve your condition. If your symptoms are not improving, you may have to seek another opinion. It is up to you to research the next provider. Most specialties—such as orthopedics—have subspecialties. The subspecialties provide an even more precise level of care for specific problems.

## Information Is Endless

If you are diagnosed with an illness or have an injury, you may be much better off than your parents and grandparents. Never before has there been such a volume of information available to everyone. Nearly every family has access to the Internet. If you do not have your own computer, public libraries are equipped with internet-ready computers for your use. There are countless books written each year covering most illness and injuries. If you cannot get to the library, you may have a friend or family member who has access to the Internet on his computer. There are also local agencies available to help individuals with disabilities. You can search in the yellow pages for various support groups for people with a similar diagnosis.

An Internet search can be as simple or as complex as you make it. Formal computer training is not necessary to search the Internet. Appendix C contains a brief list of general references on the Internet if you need a place to start. Once you begin a search for your diagnosis, you will find there may be hundreds, or even thousands, of sites from which to choose. You should avoid sites that offer only anecdotal advice (personal experience stories and conversation), such as those found in chat rooms. Search for sites that are recognized by professionals in the medical industry. Such sites may include the CDC (Centers for Disease Control), the NIH (National Institute of Health), OSHA (Occupational Safety and Health Administration) or those sites specific to the various medical specialties, such as the AAOS (American Association of Orthopedic Surgery).

You may feel more comfortable in a chat room on the Internet, but it is important to get the facts first. It is important to understand what the standards of care are for your specific illness or injury. A *standard of care* is a practice that is widely accepted in the professional community for specific diagnoses and treatment plans. It is the guide that most practitioners in a given specialty will follow. For example, if you want information about the standards of care for treating back pain, you could simply enter:

"standards of care for treatment of back pain." You will see that there are thousands of sites. Try to focus on sites set up by the leaders in healthcare. If you do not know what specialty normally would treat your condition, you can always call your primary physician and ask. Local agencies devoted to assisting individuals with disabilities can also get this information for you.

Newspapers, television and radio programs frequently offer documentaries on various diseases and injuries. The reports often provide information on the latest in treatment trends and research. They also will occasionally offer information about experimental trials that are being done at some of the larger research facilities. Do not exclude any of these sources when trying to find information. If you have above-average research, writing and reading skills, you can also search out information about the outcomes of lawsuits based on similar injuries or illnesses in your state. Oftentimes you will be able to access this information on your state's workers' compensation web site, or your state's Supreme Court website. Do not use this research to decide if you have a claim. Use it as a starting place if you have questions about how various claims are handled by your state agency. If there are several claims with similar outcomes, you may begin to notice certain patterns of care. You might also get the names of certain doctors who treat the type of injury or illness you have, and/or identify physicians who work for the insurance companies and those who support the injured or ill individuals. As you do your research, you should keep lists of questions that you want to discuss with your physician and attorney.

## Education Gives Power And Control

When you educate yourself about your illness or injury, you have power and control over your condition. You are able to make informed decisions. You will begin to understand what you can expect from your illness and injury. You will learn what usually happens along the way to recovery and what risks you might face.

Once you have all the information that you need, you will be able to make an informed decision as to whether you want to proceed with the proposed procedure or treatment plan. Oftentimes you may be in a situation that does not allow you the time to do this information-gathering. If this is the case, you will have to rely on your trust in your healthcare provider. If this is an emergency procedure or treatment, you will not have the luxury to research the plan and get another opinion. Your family or advocate should take over where you leave off. If you cannot pursue further information, someone else should make sure that the plan is appropriate for you.

If you are concerned that you may have been mistreated by a provider and wonder if you have a malpractice claim that is complicating your illness or injury, you need to do some investigating. Do an Internet search of common complications associated with your condition. Check to see if the problems that you are having are sometimes expected side-effects or risks related to your particular condition. Just be aware that there are some complications which may be unavoidable. If you cannot find the answers for yourself, you should discuss this with another physician or your lawyer. Remember that most doctors will not implicate another doctor if there is a question of malpractice. The medical community is a tightly-knit group and it is unusual that one physician will speak out against another. To get one physician to identify substandard practice by another physician, he will usually act as an expert witness, paid for by your attorney. An expert may also be hired by the defense to dispute your allegations. Unless there is a blatant issue of neglect that is obvious to the layperson, it is unlikely that one doctor will come right out and tell you another doctor made a mistake. Some communities are very small and the medical business is very limited. When one doctor implicates another doctor or healthcare provider for malpractice, it can have a very negative impact on the physician who identifies the problem. Some physicians will try to persuade a patient not to pursue a question of malpractice. They may not be truthful, even going so far as to deny there was a mistake. They might say that speaking to a lawyer will only "end up costing everyone a lot of money."

## An Objective Opinion Is Vital

You should always consider getting a second opinion. Do not leave the decisions about your care entirely to one person. If you pursue a second opinion, and the information you receive from that doctor conflicts with what you were told before, you might consider getting a third or even a fourth opinion. If your doctor or other healthcare provider ridicules or dismisses your desire to get another opinion, or says that getting another opinion would only add unnecessary additional expenses to your claim, you should interpret that to mean that you definitely should seek out another opinion. A competent physician understands the wisdom in seeking corroboration and welcomes his patients to do so. Red flags should wave if a physician stands in the way of this process. It is never appropriate for a doctor to intimidate you or threaten to discharge you from his practice if you wish to seek another opinion.

If there is any discussion about a surgical procedure—unless it is an emergency procedure—you should not sign the consent for the surgery until you have a second opinion confirming the medical necessity of this procedure. It is an arrogant, unprofessional, unethical healthcare provider who would discourage or bar this process. You want a confident physician to treat your problems, but you do not need someone who denies your right to informed consent. A second opinion may be one of the most important educational tools that you have at your disposal.

If you are going to get another opinion, you want it to be objective. Do not seek this opinion from another physician in your physician's practice or referral group. You want your second opinion to address your needs. It is unusual for a partner to speak out or advise against the treatment recommendations of another partner in his own group. It is even rarer that if a problem is identified, you will be notified about it by your physician's partner. When you look for another opinion, try to see a specialist in the same field as your doctor who can *objectively* look at whether your current treatment plan is appropriate or if there are alternative treatments which might be better. Second opinions can be found by calling other physician groups locally, or by asking others who have had similar problems as you. You can also check with larger healthcare facilities for the names and clinics of specialists outside your area.

## Check The Doctor's Record

Another important educational tool is to contact your state's professional licensing department or board of professional conduct to see if there is any record of prior complaints or lawsuits against your provider. Some states have set up Internet sites which will help you find out if your doctor has been sued previously. Most states have set up their own websites through their state health department or medical association websites. You can also try to find information on the National Practitioner Data Bank (www.npdb-hipdb.com). If you cannot find anything on the Internet, call your state medical society or Bar Association to get the name of the agency responsible for monitoring episodes of malpractice and misconduct. Your local newspaper, television or radio station may also have information if there has been a series of problems with a certain provider.

Over the past few years, there have been news articles (print and televised) which depict the plight of physicians who have to pay exorbitant malpractice premiums and who are "forced out of business" because of these premiums. If you feel you have a claim, you must pursue it, or at least discuss it with your lawyer. It is true that there are numerous malpractice suits every year which contribute to the high malpractice insurance premiums paid by physicians. However, the increases in insurance premiums do not occur without a prior claim on the physician or someone in his practice. Some physicians may belong to larger collectives who purchase insurance as a group, but the same can be said for them. The insurance companies do not usually increase premiums unless they have paid on a large claim.

## Is Your Physician Worth More Than You?

If you are the victim of medical malpractice which complicates your condition or slows your recovery, you deserve to be compensated. Future care, pain and suffering, and even loss of your ability to earn a living can cost you hundreds of thousands of dollars, if not more. If you listen to some of the lawmakers and medical groups complaining about the high medical malpractice insurance premiums affecting the earning power of physicians, you might not pursue a claim. You need to ask yourself, "Is the physician's financial well-being any more important than my own?" Where will you get the money for any needed extra care if there is no settlement? How will you pay your bills if you cannot work because of a medical mistake? Who will take care of your family's financial needs if you die from the mistake?

The patients who suffer the losses and the lawyers who represent them are often blamed for filing "frivolous" lawsuits and causing high malpractice premiums. What about the insurance industry profits and physician profits that are excluded from this picture? Insurance is a business of risk. The insurance companies gamble that they can make more money in premiums than they have to pay out to settle their claims. Medicine is a business. Insurance is a business. Malpractice claims and higher insurance premiums are part of the cost of doing business. It is uncommon to see a poor physician or insurance executive. It is not uncommon to see a person whose life has been devastated by a mistake and now cannot afford to manage his continued care.

## If You Are Accountable, You Must Be Responsible

When a person first calls a lawyer about a possible claim, the attorney is bound by the rules of his state to make sure that the claim is legitimate and not frivolous. Some lawyers will advise their clients to settle the claim for a smaller amount, to reduce the risk of a smaller award from the jury. The physician will settle in order to avoid a possible larger award by the court. There is usually some clause in the settlement that states the settlement is being made without the admission of liability. Some states call these Compromise and Release Settlements. A Compromise and Release pays the past bills associated with the claim and usually throws in some additional money to cover additional expenses. A Compromise and Release can include a clause that still requires the carrier to cover future medicals, or it may simply state that this is an all-inclusive settlement. In other words, rather than risking a possible loss in court (which would cost them more money), some carriers try to make certain claims go away. The person paying the settlement will not admit if they are responsible for the mistake. The vast majority of claims are settled before they even get to court. It might be fair to say that these claims would not be settled if there was no evidence of liability.

Insurance companies have teams of lawyers working very hard to settle claims before the cases go to court. They know that in some cases settling a claim before it goes to court can save them huge amounts of money. Defense attorneys work for the insurance companies to provide possible scenarios of what might happen if they go to court and lose. They will oftentimes try to get their clients—the insurance companies—to make an offer to make the claim go away and get rid of any future liability. Frequently they use complex documents to prepare estimates of the potential lifetime costs they might be forced to pay. They will then make an offer to you or your lawyer to settle your claim. There may be a significant difference between what they offer and what your future care might cost. They may offer a deal that sounds great to you, but represents a very small percent of what your care may actually end up costing you.

Many carriers are having Life Care Plans, Medical Cost Analyses or Medicare Set-Aside Allocations written to see what the potential future costs may be. They can use this information to meet their obligations under the Medicare system, but they also can use this information to size up their possible losses. If you have any knowledge that one of these was written, you and your lawyer should read it carefully before accepting any settlement. It is important to do your research about your illness or injury so that you understand any future care you may need. It may sound great to have an offer of $50,000 made to settle your claim, but if your future care costs will be $55,000, you will be left with bills you might not be able to pay.

There are some larger cases that do make it to the trial court. These are the cases you hear about that are tried with juries who are sympathetic to the person filing the suit and settle on a large award. But these large jury awards are the exceptions rather than the rule. There are new laws which limit the amount of awards given in some situations. For example, some states limit the amount of money that can be awarded by a jury for punitive damages. That means that the jury might award a higher payout, given as *punishment* for the mistake. In some states without caps, such an award might be in excess of a million dollars, but in states that have stricter rules, the limit for punitive damages can be significantly less.

There are certain specialties in medicine which have higher base insurance premiums; this is because these particular specialties—for example, obstetrics and gynecology or neurosurgery—are known to carry higher risks of possible complications and error rates for the physicians in those groups. It may be very important for you to know what the risks and prevalence of errors are in your particular area of care.

### Different Standards

Because a doctor has such a high level of education and expertise, she is held to a much higher standard for the work that she does. For example, a factory worker's mistakes can cause a problem with an item being produced or with the production machine; in contrast, a doctor's mistakes can seriously injure or kill a patient. It is unlikely that a factory worker will be sued for making a mistake. It is very likely that a doctor will be sued for making a mistake. As a person's education and responsibility increases and begins to have a more direct impact on the lives of others, the standards for her performance become higher, as do the penalties for her mistakes. When a doctor is accused of making a mistake, the laws are very specific when defining what a mistake is. If a doctor handles a situation one way, and a factory worker tries to handle a similar situation, the doctor and the factory worker will not be held to the same level of expectation. There are specific laws in each state which say how (or if) a doctor can be accused or sued for a mistake. There are also laws in these states which define how the doctor and her lawyer can defend that mistake. If the doctor is a general practitioner in a small community, it is likely that she will not be held to the same level of scrutiny as, say, a doctor with several additional years of specialized training who works in a larger inner-city facility.

If a patient is discharged to home early, he is supposed to be shown how to care for himself. There should be a clear plan in place, with documented patient education ensuring that the patient can take care of his problem. If the patient goes home and his wound becomes grossly infected—requiring additional surgery and hospitalization—thereby resulting in long-term disability, the patient might argue that he was not prepared or able to take care of himself. For example, he might try to blame the doctor for the infection which occurred after he arrived home by saying that the doctor should have known better than to discharge him. There are some states that allow the defense (the doctor's lawyer) to say that a reasonable person would have done things a certain way to care for himself to avoid the problem or prevent further worsening of his condition. The defense may say that the malpractice occurred because of something the patient did or did not do after he received the care. The defense may say the patient contributed to his own problems and should have a certain percent of his benefits taken away accordingly. Some states have laws that break down how much the patient contributed to the problem and how much the doctor contributed. When patients are to be held accountable for their roles in their treatment, they need to educate themselves in preventing possible complications.

### Pre-existing Complications

If you have a pre-existing medical condition (a condition which you had prior to your most current problem) which is made worse by your current illness or injury, or which is complicating your recovery, it is important to notify all of your treating providers. For example, if you are a diabetic, and you have a problem with chronic pain or a wound that is not healing on your foot, it is important to understand how the two diagnoses may be related. It is important for all of your caregivers to understand this. Learning about your medical conditions can help you understand the possible complications you might face. You may learn ways to avoid complications. It is common for a patient not to be explicitly told what the doctor feels is a common-sense thing to do. Some doctors forget that a patient is under extreme stress when they are ill or injured. When someone is under stress, she may not remember the obvious things she needs to do to take care of herself.

A pre-existing medical condition such as diabetes or poor circulation can lead to a greater risk of infection and prolonged healing time. It can contribute to additional pain. It is very important that you work to maintain control over your medical conditions, and make sure that all of your physicians work *together* to minimize the possible complications. It is not enough to see your primary physician for pre-operative medical clearance before your surgery, and then not schedule a follow-up appointment when you are discharged from the hospital.

**Infections Are On The Rise**

The rate of hospital-acquired infections is increasing. These infections are not always monitored as reportable incidences by the various state and federal health agencies. Hospitals are able to hide their statistics about these infections under the protective umbrella of "quality control" information. Recent news reports indicate that the problems with hospital-acquired infections and injuries continue to worsen. There are some statistics in October 15, 2004 issue of the *American Journal of Respiratory and Critical Care Medicine* stating that 90,000 people die every year from infections they acquired while they were in the hospital. Some consumer advocacy groups are trying to have laws passed that will make it harder for hospitals and providers to hide this information.

If you have a hospital-acquired infection, you need to have information available that will help you take care of yourself. For example, if you were not ill before you went into the hospital for an elective (non-emergency) procedure, and you developed an infection after the surgery, it would be likely that your infection is a hospital-acquired one. Some types of wound infections—such as Methicillin-Resistant Staphylococcus Aureus (MRSA, often referred to as a staph infection)—are usually only found in hospitals. If you have an infection and it is not a problem you had when you entered the hospital, you need to ask very specific questions about the infection. Many times the hospital staff or your doctors will try to skirt the issue and say it "sometimes happens" or "is not uncommon." You must persist and demand to have specific information about the infection. You need to know if it is the type of infection that will cause complications for just a few weeks, or for the rest of your life. You will need to know if your family is at risk as a result of this infection.

The research you will have to do may be difficult. You may find some of the information at the CDC or at your local health department. You may also have to request a consult with an infectious disease specialist or an epidemiologist to create a plan of care that is individualized to your needs. You will most likely need a lawyer to help you sort out the legal aspects connected to your infection. A lawyer can help you understand whether your infection is grounds for a lawsuit. The lawyer will do everything he can to help determine if the hospital staff did everything they could—including following their own policies—to reduce your exposure to infection. He will also make sure that the procedures used to care for you were like those used by other professionals in similar situations. Finally, he will have to identify a specific mistake that caused your infection. This is when your explicit recordkeeping or your advocate's recordkeeping will come into play. If you can identify the specific names of your caregivers and times and dates when you noticed them not wash their hands or do something else that you felt might expose you to an infection; it will be helpful when your lawyer is trying to sort out the details of your case. Because of the variables related to every individual situation, there is no way to know who is liable and to what degree until a thorough review of your care has been completed.

Even though a physician might say there is a risk of infection when going over the risks and benefits of a procedure or treatment, it does not mean that you must just accept it if an infection develops. There are some infections that are known to happen with certain procedures. It is up to the doctor and hospital staff to ensure that you do not develop an infection or suffer additional injury because of their negligence.

If you are told you have an infection while you are still in the hospital, of course you will not be able to research the facts around that type of infection. Your family or advocate can do so for you. If the doctor comes to your room and tells you that you will need antibiotics for an infection, make her write down on a piece of paper what type of infection it is. This will help your family find the information they need to make sure that you get the appropriate care. Acinetobacter baumannii, MRSA and VRE, C. Difficile and Pseudomonas aeruginosa are some examples of hospital-acquired infections. Most hospital-acquired infections can be treated with antibiotics or combinations of antibiotics; however, for some patients with compromised immune systems, or who are critically ill related to their underlying illness, a hospital-acquired infection can be deadly.

## Make Them Wash Their Hands!

You need to educate yourself about the number one infection control prevention in this country that still is not being universally practiced. It can protect you at home, work, in the hospital, wherever you go. You must *insist* that each and every caretaker who approaches you washes her hands. In the hospital or in a private office—whether to make the bed, do a dressing change, check your blood pressure or listen to your heart and lungs—all providers *must* wash their hands before they perform any examination or other care-giving task. You cannot control breaks in the sterilization procedures in the operating room. You *can* insist that physicians, nurses and other staff wash their hands and practice universal precautions to prevent infections such as Methicillin Resistant Staphylococcus Aureus (MRSA) or Vancomycin Resistant Enterococcus (VRE).

## If You Develop An Infection At Home

If you are home and you develop a post-operative wound infection, call your surgeon immediately. Depending on the severity of the infection and the additional care it may require, you may want to consult with an attorney on how best to proceed. Unless people start demanding better care, problems will remain hidden by the healthcare business industry. If infections were to be generally accepted as a routine part of your care, the institutions and government agencies would not devote so much time and money to trying to erase the problem and shroud the results under non-discoverable quality umbrellas. Millions of people are infected every year. Billions are spent trying to treat those infections.

## Do Not Ignore Pain

Pain is an expected result of certain procedures. However, pain should not be ignored. Pain should be treated and the cause identified. Neither acute pain (the kind you have right after an accident or surgery) nor chronic pain (the kind that goes on for weeks and years afterwards) should be something with which you simply to learn to live. As healing occurs, pain should improve. Some pre-existing medical conditions such as diabetes can cause pain to worsen and persist over time. In some diabetics, the damage to nerves caused by the diabetes can make pain worsen. But do not assume that your pain is due to a pre-existing problem until a physician has ruled out all other causes of your pain. If your pain is worse than pain you have had in the past, let your physician know. Do some research to find out how much pain is normally expected. If you are a person who usually has a high pain tolerance and now you require more narcotics because your pain is worsening, you need to discuss this with your physician.

## Calling The Doctor

When you call your doctor you will probably speak with the receptionist or secretary. She will take a message and pass it on to your doctor. The secretary or receptionist should not be judgmental. She should not be making a diagnosis regarding your complaints of pain. The office staff should not be telling you what to do before they speak to the doctor. Medical professionals should be the only people prescribing your care. A secretary can relay a message but should never offer medical advice.

Diagnoses should not be offered over the phone. Sometimes doctors will train their staff and provide them with certain guidelines that allow the nurses to add extra patients to the office schedule that day. If you call and are discouraged from coming in to see the doctor and you feel it is urgent that you or your loved one be seen, insist on an appointment. If they refuse to see you, go to the emergency room or urgent care clinic. If you feel comfortable with the advice you are given from the staff without your doctor's input, you should do what feels right for you. Remember, only the doctor, an advanced practice registered nurse (nurse practitioner) or physician assistant can make a diagnosis and prescribe care. If you accept care from a nurse or secretary without the benefit of the doctor's input, you may suffer further complications from the misdiagnosis of your problem.

It may take a few hours for the physician or her nurse to get back to you with what you need to do. However, do not wait a whole day without an answer. If you cannot tolerate the pain or other symptoms you have, ask for an urgent appointment with the doctor, or ask for a referral to the emergency room. Many insurances—whether they are private health plans, workers' compensation or managed care plans—require referrals to the emergency room. Some do not. It is a good idea to have a referral from your physician. If your doctor or his office staff call the emergency room and let them know that you are on the way, it helps the emergency room prepare for your arrival—especially if you have an urgent problem, or complicated medical history. Do not hesitate to call the office more than once if you feel that your complaints are not being addressed. If your pain is not relieved, you need to insist on seeing the physician.

## Not All Patients Are Drug-Seeking

Some doctors are very skeptical of a patient who complains of a lot of pain. Some doctors have been burned in the past by patients lying about their pain and medication use. They may believe that after a certain period of time their patients should not need to use narcotics to manage their pain. Some emergency rooms and healthcare providers actually have lists of patients whom they believe are drug-seeking. Unfortunately a few people who are drug-seekers have ruined it for many people who have a legitimate need for pain-management medication.

There are some doctors who may misdiagnose a patient's ongoing complaints of pain. Their minds are closed to the possibility that not all patients can tolerate equal amounts of pain. This may cause additional harm to the patient. For example, Barrie continued to talk to his physician and her staff about his terrible pain. Barrie was not assertive enough, and was easily intimidated by the hurried, brusque demeanor of the doctor and the condescending protectiveness of the secretary taking messages at the front desk. The physician and her secretary actually suggested to Barrie that there was some concern that he was looking for drugs. Barrie became very upset and began to doubt himself. He wondered if he really did have a problem, or if it was something he was imagining. Finally Barrie insisted the doctor do some additional testing. The doctor discovered the surgery had not worked the way it should, and Barrie needed additional surgery.

If your doctor is not listening, be persistent until she does, or find another one who will. Not all people who have complaints of severe, chronic pain are narcotic-seeking.

## The Patient Is Not Always Wrong!

After several months of suffering and complaining about uncontrolled pain, Rachel went for her follow-up appointment with her surgeon, and her husband, Isaac, accompanied her. Isaac explained what his wife's suffering was like and how it affected everything she tried to do. The doctor appeared to be only partially interested, again expressing concern that Rachel enjoyed being home and was beginning to develop an unhealthy dependence on medication. He then suggested that Rachel was using the medications for reasons other than pain management, while getting paid by workers' compensation to stay home. Isaac became irate. He suggested that the physician was incompetent for ignoring his wife's complaints. Finally, the physician agreed to consider that there might be a complication that had been overlooked. When Rachel's husband suggested that his lawyer would contact the physician to see why something had not been done, the physician reluctantly agreed to order some x-rays. (Rachel had not had any x-rays or other tests done for the several months she had been complaining of the terrible pain.)

Imagine the doctor's surprise when the x-ray revealed that there was a problem with one of the parts in Rachel's newly-replaced artificial joint. The pain was not a figment of Rachel's imagination, nor was it a way to obtain more narcotic medications and be paid to stay home. Thus these several months later—after months of unnecessary pain and suffering—Rachel was faced with another joint replacement, more extensive surgery and another spell of rehabilitation. She finally went to another doctor for a second opinion. Rachel was told that if the problem with the artificial joint had been discovered sooner, she could have had aggressive physical therapy which would have helped her avoid the additional surgery. It would have also helped her avoid several months of pain and suffering and embarrassment from being told that she was enjoying the medications and staying out of work.

### Be Persistent!

If you have a persistent problem, it is up to you to pursue it. If there is an obvious problem such as the one Rachel experienced, only your persistence will help the physician search further. He should know that if he does not, his liabilities increase: First, for poor care in failing to diagnose the actual problem; second, for failing to listen to the patient; and third, for failing to provide adequate medication and care to control the pain.

It can be difficult to accept human error, and our physicians and nurses are human; but it is nearly impossible to accept an error when the perpetrator tries to somehow imply that patients are lying or causing the problem. Medicine is not an exact science. It is a scientific art practiced by humans, and humans make errors. Anyone can make a mistake, but when a physician does not listen to his patient, it is not a mistake, it is negligence. If your physician is not listening and your complaints fall on deaf or uncaring ears, find another physician.

### Know What To Expect

Do not just give up control of your life to someone who swore an oath to protect and do no harm, and who can change the course of your life completely. If you are faced with the possibility of a surgical procedure in the near future, you must do your homework. Research everything you can find about the procedure. Investigate the risks associated with the procedure, as well as what the past outcomes and successes have been. Find out what the issues are for others you know who have had similar problems. If after all of your research you still have questions, and need additional information about how your physician might handle the various issues you have identified, make sure to meet with him again to answer your questions before heading to the operating room.

### Heading Off A Problem

Ralph had a past history of alcohol and substance abuse. He was to undergo a rather routine surgical procedure to repair a ligament in his knee, and had no other medical conditions that were anticipated to complicate the post-operative course. Ralph's surgeon, Dr. Smith, was well-known in the community to be very conservative regarding his prescription of post-operative narcotics. Dr. Smith did not believe in using a lot of narcotics to control pain. He believed that over-the-counter medications should be just as effective. His patients were very pleased with his exceptional surgical abilities, but many were very dissatisfied with the amount of pain they seemed to have after their surgery. Ralph set up a meeting with Dr. Smith to discuss what he could expect after his discharge from the hospital and how his post-operative pain would be managed.

Ralph's history of alcohol and drug abuse could have seriously compromised his pain control in what was a routine procedure with a very high incidence of post-operative pain. The treatment of post-operative pain became the major problem to be anticipated. If Ralph and his doctor had not had a frank discussion about his problems with drugs and alcohol before his surgery, Ralph could have had a significant problem with post-operative pain management. By addressing the problem with his doctor, Ralph was able to have an individualized pain management plan in place before he went to the hospital. Dr. Smith's staff understood that there were exceptional issues with Ralph's condition, and the covering physicians in Dr. Smith's practice were less reluctant to reorder medications or see Ralph when he called with a problem. Ralph's physician understood that Ralph was less likely to get the same relief from a medication as another patient without a prior abuse history might receive. His doctor knew that Ralph's past history might make him less able to tolerate discomfort without the benefit of stronger medications. He realized that in some cases, patients who do not have a past history of drug use require less medication than someone like Ralph. This is not always true, but for this particular patient it was.

Some patients, no matter what their past history, do not tolerate any discomfort and need more medications than others in similar situations. This is why it is so important for doctors to have frank discussions with their patients. If your doctor does not bring this up with you, you should. It is very important that your doctor knows how you respond to pain before a scheduled procedure. If you are someone who has never had an injury or illness and you have a high tolerance for discomfort, let your physician know this as well. Some patients refuse to take medications for pain for religious or cultural reasons. Make sure your doctor knows about any such preference. He may be able to prescribe alternative therapies that might help reduce some of your discomfort. These might include visualization or biofeedback training, self-hypnosis or massage. If your procedure is elective, take the time to research your options. If you are concerned about a problem that you have—whether it is related to pain management, symptoms that do not seem to be addressed, or other complications—you must address it directly with your physician. If he is unwilling to discuss your problem with you, it might be time to consider finding another physician.

## Laws Can Impact Pain Management

Pain can be a normal response to an injury or illness, but severe pain that is not relieved may not be normal. Pain management has been so poorly addressed in the past by doctors and healthcare providers that recent legislation has been passed to ensure that patients' concerns are addressed. Educate yourself on the various laws enacted in the last few years that give you the right to adequate pain control. Physicians are caught between a rock and a hard place when it comes to dealing with pain. On the one hand, they have federal rules and regulations that outline patients' rights for pain control. On the other hand, physicians are scrutinized like bugs under a microscope by state and federal regulators who want to ensure that they do not prescribe too many narcotic pain medications. Some doctors may have high levels of tolerance for pain, or have never had the misfortune to have severe pain. Some doctors simply do not believe that anything can be as painful as some patients describe.

When an attending surgeon meets with a patient to obtain consent for a surgical procedure, the surgeon has an obligation to discuss, in detail, all aspects of the surgery and what the patient can expect. This discussion should include what will happen before *and* after the surgery. A discussion about pain management should be part of the consent procedure. If a patient knows that she has problems with chronic pain, these issues should be addressed before the consent is signed. It is not enough to assume that your physician will provide adequate pain management if you do not discuss his policies in advance. As a nurse who has witnessed hundreds of consents, I can tell you that the issue of pain management or post-operative care is rarely addressed by the patient or the surgeon. When an individualized pain-management plan is in place a patient can be assured that the surgeon is interested in doing what is best for the patient. A surgeon can alleviate problems for his staff (and covering physicians in his absence) when a plan is in place prior to the patient calling for a refill of her prescription.

## The Physician Needs To Know

It is not only important to educate yourself, but—as with Ralph—it is sometimes necessary to educate the physician and his staff. Do not assume that your surgeon will read or pay attention to what is in your chart. Given the volume of patients he sees every day, it is unlikely that he would remember every detail or problem with every one of his patients. The surgeon may have read the previous medical records, but he may not have identified the degree of the potential problem that could surface with this procedure. Past patients might not have had serious problems with narcotics or chronic pain, or the physician only skimmed the records and really did not believe that the proposed procedure would exacerbate any pre-existing problems.

It can be very frustrating if you go to the doctor, ensure he has your records, fill out several very long forms, and he never reads them. If the physician cannot take the time to read a few medical records, it may make you wonder if he will actually have any time for you if a problem develops. If you have a problem, or if you have more questions, make sure to have these addressed *before* you proceed with the treatment or procedure. If the physician or provider is not willing to meet with you for any reason, postpone the procedure (if possible) until you resolve the issue. If your procedure is not urgent and you feel that you are getting the run-around from the doctor, consider seeking another opinion to see if your concerns are valid and could be handled in a different way.

### Informed Consent Is Your Right

You will be asked to sign a consent form before a procedure. When you sign the consent, you are stating that the physician has answered all of your questions and you agree to have the procedure. Informed consent is the legal and ethical right of every patient. It gives you control over what happens to your body. Informed consent also extends to the legal and the ethical duty of the physician to involve the patient in healthcare decisions. You cannot make an informed choice without all of the information. This does not pertain just to the procedure itself, but also to what you can expect after the procedure.

### Your Advocate Needs To Know

Obviously, if you are taken to the emergency department at the time of your injury or illness, you do not have the luxury of the time to educate yourself. However, it is important that someone representing you do the work. If you cannot speak for yourself, it falls to your family or advocate to give the consent for the care you need. This places the burden of knowledge on them. Once you are home and able to function, you can take a look back at what happened and look ahead to review your plan. When you give your consent in non-emergent situations, be sure to identify who your advocate, health care proxy or health care power of attorney is. A health care proxy is a person whom you designate to be able to make all of your healthcare decisions (with some restrictions, if you choose) if you are unable to do so. Your health care proxy, advocate or health care power of attorney can be a family member, friend or even your lawyer. Before you complete the papers identifying a proxy, be sure to discuss this fully with the person you designate.

If you have a health care proxy, advocate or health care power of attorney, make sure that your physician, the hospital and everyone involved in your care has a copy of the agreement or proxy form. Health Care Proxy forms can be downloaded from multiple Internet websites. Just go to the search bar and type in *health care proxy forms*. You can specifically add your state's name to the search for a more specific form. You can also pick them up at your doctor's office, the library or the hospital. *Every* person over the age of 18 should have a health care proxy on file. Be sure to keep a copy of your form in your binder with all of your other documents. Some people will place proxy forms in safe deposit boxes, which is absolutely the last place they should be. They should be easily accessible to the person who is your advocate, not locked away in a bank vault.

### Paying For Medicine

Another issue often forgotten when patients are educating themselves about a possible upcoming procedure is the need for special equipment or medications post-operatively. It is not uncommon to hear patients say that they expect everything should be paid for by the carrier. This is correct in some cases.

However, without adequate preparation, the patient may be discharged with several prescriptions that will be needed as soon as they get home. A big problem for patients immediately after discharge can be their first stop at the pharmacy. Skyrocketing drug costs can leave the patient feeling worse than the actual injury or illness. If there is time, educate yourself by finding out what types of medications will be used; then check to see if your prescriptions will be covered by your insurance. Find out how much will be paid by the insurance and how much you are expected to pay. Find out if you have to pay out of your pocket and then wait for reimbursement (as with most traditional insurance plans). The physician may not be able to tell you exactly what you will be prescribed, but you can get an idea of what types of medications you might need.

Many carriers have agreements with pharmacy providers throughout the country that will allow a credit type of system that allows you to pick up your medications or equipment needs without having to pay cash up-front. In this system, the patient does not have to pay the pharmacy and then submit his bill to the carrier for reimbursement. When a patient has to pay huge costs up-front and endure carrier delays in reimbursement, it can create financial difficulties. This financial burden can contribute to overall stress, which in turn can delay the healing process. Some patients will not fill prescriptions for this very reason. It is nearly impossible to pay a couple of hundred dollars for a prescription when your workers' compensation benefits or disability insurance benefits are only a couple of hundred dollars a week, or have not even begun yet.

## Be A Smart Consumer

If you feel that you need a new physician, follow your instincts. It is not uncommon for patients to continue to see a physician because they like him and are reluctant to change. They may have known the physician for years. It is wonderful to have a good rapport and past history with a provider. However, if your physician is not aware of current trends and treatment protocols, you may be in for some trouble if your condition is complex. You need to continue to educate yourself throughout the process. Never stop learning. You are your own best advocate. If you cannot look out for yourself, find someone who can. Do not assume that you are anyone's number one priority. Healthcare is a business just like any other, and you must learn to be a smart consumer. You are not buying a new car; you are hiring someone to help you through your health crisis. Most people spend more energy and time shopping for and arguing over the cost of a new car than they do over their own health care.

## Cultural Beliefs Can Affect Your Care

Another point to consider is the role cultural and traditional values will play in your recovery. It is important for you to let the physician know if there are certain beliefs you have that may impact how you receive your care. For example, Jehovah's Witnesses refuse to accept blood transfusions, even if it means life or death. If you are dealing with a language barrier, ask to have an interpreter present. If an interpreter is needed in a hospital or other place that receives funding or provides governmental services, the hospital or other agency will pay for this service. If an interpreter is needed for a workers' compensation, Medicare or disability claimant, the insurance will usually pay the interpreter fees. (If you do not have any insurance, you are encouraged to contact your local social services department for assistance.) These issues must be addressed if your recovery is to proceed.

## In Summary

Remember some of the key points to educating yourself. You will need the answers to the following questions:
- What is my diagnosis?
- What does it mean for me?
- What is the prognosis?
- Will I be bothered by this for the rest of my life?

- What are my treatment options?
- What are the side effects of my treatment?
- Are there any alternative treatments?
- Is this physician or healthcare provider the most knowledgeable and appropriate to coordinate my care? Who can best treat my problem?
- How will this affect the rest of my life/work/family?
- Who can I look to for help with ongoing problems?

One final point to remember is that if you cannot get in to see your doctor and you are having troubles, you should go to your local emergency room or urgent care clinic. This is not always an efficient way to manage your care, but for some people it is the only way to be evaluated when there is a pressing problem. Some doctors are so overbooked that they have no room on their schedules for any additions. It is not uncommon for there to be too few physicians and too many patients in a community, resulting in resources so far stretched that the only alternative for emergent care becomes the local emergency room. The emergency room becomes an extension of the doctor's office. This practice overwhelms the emergency rooms and drives costs up further, but until doctors' offices can keep up with the demand it seems to be the only alternative.

If you find yourself in this situation, be prepared for a long wait at the hospital, unless your condition is life-threatening or requires urgent attention. Emergency rooms do not operate on a first-come, first-served basis. They take the sickest, most unstable patients first. Your condition—although it might seem urgent to you that day—might not be urgent in comparison to the general emergency room population. If you are unsure about whether you should go to the emergency room or the urgent care clinic, you probably should go to the emergency room and let them assess you and refer you on if appropriate. There are too many symptoms that require emergency room care, even though they seem like they could be handled in the urgent care facility. These can be affected by the patient's age and overall health status. To provide a list of illnesses or injuries that should be treated in the urgent care clinic instead of the emergency room would be inappropriate and—for some patients—dangerous.

## Things To Remember

- Do not assume anyone knows everything.
- If someone tells you they know everything... run.
- If his mind is closed to new ideas, find someone whose is open.
- Review all reports for accuracy. Are they really referring to you?
- If the report is inaccurate, seek to have it corrected immediately.
- Find out who employs the doctor.
- Search for *factual* information from as many sources as you can.
- Take control of the situation and address the questions you have.
- Getting a second opinion is vital; an objective opinion can save your life.
- Check out the provider's record and work history—make sure he is not practicing without a license, and has a clean history.
- Decide that your health is worth more than your provider's bank account.
- Do not hide pre-existing problems—learn how they impact your current condition.
- Do not let your complaints of pain be ignored.
- Make everyone wash their hands.
- Understand to what you are consenting.
- Let your provider know if you have cultural beliefs which impact your care.

- Do I trust others too freely?
- Am I following orders and prescriptions without asking "Why?" and "What are they for?"
- Why am I taking this or doing this?
- How long do I need to take or do this?
- What should I expect as a result of this plan?
- How will it help?
- How can it hurt me?
- What should I do if there is a problem?
- Will this interfere with other treatments that I may need?
- Have you shared this plan with all of my other providers to avoid interactions or complications?
- How can I get a copy of my record?
- Does my doctor have a release to provide access to and share my health information with my advocate, health care proxy or attorney?
- Have I obtained copies of all of my records to date and filed them in my binder? Have I read these records to verify they are mine? If I have questions, have they been brought to the attention of my provider, and if so, have they been answered?
- Which state agency or professional licensure agency oversees my providers? Do I know how to reach them if there is a problem?
- Have I noted to whom I have talked, why I talked to them and the date and time so that I can refer back to this for future questions?
- For whom does my doctor work? Is he self-employed, part of a private corporation or a member of a managed care network?
- Does my doctor have a contract with my employer? Is my doctor or provider watching out for my interests, or someone else's?
- Have I had a second (or third or fourth) opinion yet? Do I understand, if there is a discrepancy, *what* it is, *why* it is, and what the alternative treatment options are?
- Do I understand what has been said to me?
- How is my provider's professional record? Does he have certifications in the appropriate specialty for me to have the best care for my condition? Is his license current?
- Have I been completely honest about my past medical history, medication use and treatments which I have had?
- Am I at risk of further injury, complications or infection due to poor care or improper hygiene from my providers?
- Has my provider addressed my pain and my complaints adequately? Do I feel that my provider is hearing my concerns? Am I being treated as an individual?
- Do I have special cultural or religious beliefs that I need to share with my advocate and providers to ensure that my care is tailored to incorporate those special needs?
- Have I identified my advocate/health care proxy/power of attorney to assist me through this process?

**6**

## Past Medical History

We have all heard the saying that the past can come back to haunt us. In healthcare this may be particularly true. Most people do not realize how much what happened to them several years ago can affect what happens to them today and tomorrow. It is not uncommon to forget to mention that little problem you had when you were just a child, but it might be that particular problem that complicates your recovery now.

Lisa had several kidney infections as a child, and now has an injured back. Dr. Wells, the orthopedic surgeon treating Lisa's back injury, has prescribed several medications to treat the inflammation and control the pain. The multiple medications Lisa is taking all have warnings about the possible problems that can occur when the medications filter through the kidneys. She never told Dr. Wells about her past kidney problems, and he had no reason to worry about the potential complications that could arise when a patient has decreased kidney function. Dr. Wells did not call Lisa's primary physician to inquire about any potential kidney problems. Just imagine Dr. Wells' and Lisa's horror when the medications caused her kidneys to fail. Lisa was required to go on dialysis and eventually have a kidney transplant—all because of a back injury coupled with a failure to communicate about a past problem.

Unfortunately, Lisa lived in a state which apportioned (allocate a specific percentage of your current problem to previous problems) malpractice settlements based on prior problems. This meant that Lisa's settlement and insurance benefits were significantly reduced because of the pre-existing kidney disease. Patients should never presume that they know what is and what is not important to tell their doctors, especially when it comes to their past history and current situation.

### Reduced Benefits And Pre-existing Problems

Regardless of the type of insurance that you have for your injury or illness, you will need to clarify with your carrier or state agency how any pre-existing medical problems will affect your claim. There are some states which apportion and/or deny or reduce payments for a pre-existing problem. For example, if you are working and have a history of a ten-year-old back injury, and now (working for a new company) sustain another back injury which requires surgery, the carrier may apportion the amount of their responsibility to the claim. The carrier in this case may say that they are 50% responsible. You will need to speak with the individual carrier to determine the laws and specific equations used to formulate the percent of covered liability. If they apportion the claim, you may sustain an unexpected financial burden. This may be simply related to the medical costs of the claim, or it may affect everything, including your weekly compensation check and any permanent disability settlement that you might receive.

Some companies do database screens to check for past claims. There are national companies who have listings of all claims which people in this country have settled. For example, if you had a car accident eighteen years ago and had a severe back injury for which you sued and won a settlement, you might be surprised to learn that this settlement information was entered into a national data bank. The adjustor on your current claim only needs to do a search to find out about your past claims. Some adjustors will use this information to determine what they will or will not approve when it comes to your current claim. If they think that your current injury or illness is directly related to your past claim, it is possible that your current claim will be denied. You will then have to prove that although you had the prior condition, this current problem is unrelated. In the case of a denial due to a supposed pre-existing condition, you will most likely need the services of a lawyer to appeal and fight for benefits to cover your current claim.

## Not All Plans Have Pre-existing Exemptions

Some states accept the claimants "as they are." These states recognize that there may be a pre-existing medical problem or injury which has been worsened by, or contributes to, your current injury or illness. Because of the rules and regulations adopted by these states, they accept that this is part of the current claim and cover the costs of the claim. You can imagine that this can contribute significantly to the costs of workers' compensation in those states and therefore, many states are addressing these issues and amending their rules and regulations accordingly.

Although they are not all-inclusive, and can be new or acute problems, some examples of pre-existing problems are heart disease, diabetes, prior injuries, lung disease and arthritis.

## Waiting Periods And Excluded Diagnoses

If your injury or illness is not work-related, you will need to check with your individual insurance carrier to determine if any pre-existing conditions may affect your claim. This is usually an issue when a new policy is issued, especially if you have not been covered by another insurance plan from your previous employer. You will need to verify this with the carrier. The Health Insurance Portability and Accountability Act of 1996 (HIPAA) was passed to provide rights and protection for participants and beneficiaries of group health plans. (For more information on HIPAA you can go to www.cms.hhs.gov/hipaa.) Many carriers will have lists of diagnoses which they exclude from coverage. These may or may not be pre-existing conditions; regardless, the carriers have chosen not to cover them. This means that if you have a condition which is pre-existing and is excluded from coverage, or for which there is a specific waiting period for coverage, you will need to comply with the policy restrictions. This is not to say that you cannot seek treatment for the problem, but you will have to pay for the costs of the treatment out of your own pocket.

All diagnoses are given specific codes and all billing is processed using computers. Computer programs have been designed to identify the excluded diagnoses and automatically reject payment for those claims. You may have little chance on appeal, but it is worth following the entire appeals process outlined in your insurance handbook. If you receive a bill stating that it was rejected or denied, and you call the customer service number listed on the bill, do not be surprised if you are told only that the bill has been denied and you must pay. It is unlikely that you will be told how to appeal the denial and what the process can entail. An appeal can be long and very frustrating, but it is important that you follow the process step-by-step to make sure that you are not denied on a technicality in the process.

## Lifetime Benefit Limits

As time goes on, medicine is able to identify more chronic conditions. These are not just limited to our older population; children and young adults can also suffer from chronic conditions. If you or your child suffers from a chronic ailment, it will be important for you to understand how your carrier will cover the treatments for this condition. There are some carriers who set limits on the amount of treatment that can be provided. For example, there may be preset dollar limits or limited number of treatments allowed for certain types of care. If you need care beyond these limits you may have to pay out-of-pocket costs. As there is no universal health insurance, the amount of covered care you receive can be very different from another person with the same medical needs who has an insurance policy with more liberal (or non-existent) policy limits. Check with your carrier. Whether you are being treated for a work-related illness or injury or not, it is important that you understand what the financial limits to your care will be.

## Future Benefits

When you have an illness or injury, it is hoped that you will recover at some point, or at least that the condition will no longer be an acute problem. At that point, it becomes a past medical problem. You will need to understand if your pre-existing condition excludes you from coverage now, or after a specific waiting period. You will also need to understand how current treatment of that condition can impact future care. If you receive a certain treatment regime now, you will need to understand the implications for the future should you need similar treatment at a later time. For example, if the policy limit is twenty visits over the lifetime of the patient, and the visits are all used up, what happens should the problem occur again in the future?

If this is a workers' compensation injury, what happens in the future if you have more problems? What happens if you need more treatment in a few years? Who pays for any future care you might need once your claim has settled? Is there a clause in your settlement or in your insurance contract stating that you are responsible for your future care, or did the agreement say that the carrier will be responsible for all future care? What happens if you are out of work again for the same problem—will you receive weekly compensation benefits to cover your lost wages if you returned to work? What if you never return to work and your doctor says that you should be entitled to temporary total disability payments? These are all questions that you need to address now.

When you try to find the answers to these questions, you may think of a several more. Be sure to write them down. As you learned earlier, if you talk to someone, make sure you have his name and the time and date of your conversation—especially if it relates to a specific benefit or coverage question. If possible, you should address your questions in a letter. If you receive a letter in response it is even better for your records. Should there be a challenge later on, you can refer to the letter as proof of previous discussions. If you have to rely on notes about your verbal discussions, the validity of your recollections may be challenged; however, the person with whom you spoke might also have made a note in his case notes or claims summary notes about your conversation. You should always ask for a copy of any case notes and other information regarding your claim.

### *Things To Remember*

- Pre-existing medical conditions may reduce your benefits.
- Not all insurance plans have pre-existing exclusions.
- Some pre-existing conditions may be covered after a waiting period.
- Some benefits have lifetime limits and restrictions.
- Failure to disclose information can lead to complications in your care or fraudulent insurance claims (a criminal offense).

### *Questions You Need To Ask*

- What pre-existing medical problems do I have?
- Have I told my providers about my past medical history?
- If I have pre-existing problems, how will they affect the outcome of my current claim?
- Am I subject to financial obligations related to my pre-existing condition?
- Do I have a waiting period before my pre-existing condition is covered?
- Have I exhausted my lifetime benefits? Does my policy have lifetime limits?
- If I have exhausted lifetime benefits, what other options are available to cover my healthcare needs?
- Have I contacted local social service agencies to help with these problems?

# 7

## *Retaining An Attorney*

*T*urn on the television any evening and you can usually see at least one or two ads for law firms or lawyers talking about the pitfalls of dealing with insurance companies. These firms spend thousands of dollars trying to get your business after you have an accident. You are wise to investigate all your options. It never hurts to call.

### Request An Initial Consultation

Throughout this book, you are advised about certain instances in which you should contact an attorney. Most lawyers will discuss your situation with you prior to agreeing to take your case. This is called an initial consultation. This initial consultation will usually be free of charge. You may be able to accomplish this discussion of the details of your case via a simple phone call with the attorney. He should be able to tell you from this information exchange if you would benefit from legal representation. If your claim is complex, you may need to have a formal appointment to review it, especially if it has been going on for a long time. The purpose of this initial consultation is to help the lawyer decide if your case has any merit or legal standing. There has been much talk recently about "frivolous" lawsuits. When a lawyer does an initial screen of your case he can tell you, based on experience, whether or not you have a case that can stand up to the challenges of the court system.

When you sustain an injury or illness—whether related to your work, or the fault of another person—it is up to you to decide if you want to contact an attorney. In most cases, especially if it is a complicated injury or illness, or if you are going to be recovering for an extended period, you should set up an initial consultation with a lawyer who specializes in your type of claim. For example, if you have a work-related injury you will want a lawyer who specializes in workers' compensation law. If you are injured as the result of the actions of another party—such as a car accident or slip and fall on someone else's property—you will want a lawyer who specializes in negligence or personal injury. If you have a claim for disability or workers' compensation benefits which was denied, you will want to call a lawyer who specializes in this type of appeal.

### Negligent Employers

If you believe that your accident or illness is due to an obvious hazard which your employer failed to rectify, speak to an attorney. Workers' compensation is intended to be a no-fault system; it protects an employer from being sued by an employee who is injured or becomes ill while performing the duties of his job. However, if your employer is liable for or contributed to your injury, you may be able to collect more on your claim. If your employer broke a state or federal law or rule which contributed to your condition, it may be possible for you to file a claim directly against your employer. This is very complicated and will require an attorney very familiar with the laws pertaining to your line of work. For example, if you are an ironworker, you will want an attorney who is familiar with construction law as opposed to medical malpractice. You may need a lawyer who specializes in both. If you can provide detailed information to your lawyer about specific workplace hazards, he should be able to help you determine if there is another claim that can be filed.

## Lawyers Are Specialists, Too

Each area of law is specialized. Each attorney has his own field of expertise. When you first consider whether or not to contact an attorney, you will need to decide what type of claim you have. As with medicine, attorneys have specialty practices as well. Some have general law practices, but many have very specific areas of practice. You may know of attorneys locally who have assisted family or friends in similar circumstances. Whomever you choose, first be sure that your attorney has a strong reputation for his area of practice. If you are not sure about where to find an attorney who will meet your needs for a particular claim, call a lawyer referral service. Most states have lawyer referral services that can be found in the business section of the phone directory, or by contacting your state or local Bar Association.

## Who Is At Fault?

Attorneys in your state are aware of the various types of liability and can expertly counsel you in how to proceed. They can tell you if you can file a claim against another individual, or business (such as your employer) or manufacturer. Any question you have about other factors which may have directly or indirectly contributed to your current condition should be discussed with an attorney. Different types of liabilities—such as product liability, employer negligence or medical malpractice—are usually regulated by the state in which the offense occurred.

## Medical Malpractice Complicates Claims

Occasionally when a person is being treated for an injury or illness, he may suffer further misfortune if he is the victim of a medical mistake. If you feel that your physician or other healthcare provider has caused additional injury, or contributed to a worsening of your symptoms, you may also be able to file a medical malpractice claim. If you are in this situation, it may be difficult to prove that incorrect treatment worsened your condition; but with a thorough review of your condition and the documentation regarding your claim, a skilled attorney can help you sort this out.

## Product Liability Complicates Claims

If you believe that your illness or injury is due to the failure of a product or piece of equipment, discuss this with your attorney. This is especially important if you know of others in your workplace or neighborhood who have been injured using the same, or similar, equipment. A product liability claim may also become part of your current workers' compensation or disability claim. For example, if you are using a piece of equipment around your house and it breaks, causing an injury and disability, you may be able to collect on a product liability claim. A skilled lawyer can tell you if you have a claim or not. You may have to do some research to find out if there have been other injuries. Say you were injured using an electrical appliance; you might find this information through research on the Internet just by typing in the words "injuries from" followed by the name of whatever appliance caused your injury.

You will need to know if the injuries you received were an isolated event, or if they are consistent with a pattern of problems that have not been recognized by the manufacturer. If there are others who have had the same problems from a piece of equipment, and you can find supporting documentation in your research, this will help your attorney strengthen your claim and put together a legal case on your behalf. Most lawyers who specialize in product liability have a reference file of information regarding equipment found to contribute to injuries. If your issue is with a piece of equipment not already part of your lawyer's files, the more information you can provide to him, the better.

## Legal Experts Coordinate The Legal Issues

Whether your claim is for a work-related injury, an illness or condition related to the malfunction or a breakdown in environmental work standards, or if you are hurt on the job because of a product malfunction, you should at least review the events surrounding the claim with an attorney. You may be told that you do not have a claim; or, you may have the ability to file a claim, which will cover additional medical costs either directly or indirectly related to your condition. If you have an injury to a body part, you seek care from an expert physician who specializes in helping you get well. Let an expert in the law help you coordinate your legal claim.

The legal system is extremely complex, with specific forms and deadlines and practice protocols. A failure to follow the specific requirements can negate or cancel any chance you might have to win your claim. Lawyers know the processes and timelines. Let them manage this for you to help ensure your claim is successful.

## Before You Talk To Anyone

Should you have a question about other types of liability, and feel that there are other issues which may impact your claim, you should speak with an attorney *before* you address your concerns with your employer or carrier. This is especially true if you feel there is the possibility that your carrier or employer will try to talk you out of seeking legal counsel. They may feel that they will have less financial responsibility to you if there is not an attorney involved. Once an attorney has taken the initial information regarding the events surrounding your claim, she will be able to advise you on how to proceed. She will be very specific about with whom you should speak regarding your case. She will advise you on what you should say when you are asked about the specifics of your claim. Attorneys cannot tell you how to answer questions in court, but they can advise you on what you should or should not discuss with family, friends and coworkers. The most important advice that you will receive is this: If you are talking to anyone about your claim, it is vital that your words and actions be truthful. Do not embellish or exaggerate anything. A thorough investigation will uncover any such false claims or statements, and those findings could end any chance of a claim.

## The Advertisements Are True

If you are like millions of television viewers in this country, you have seen the advertisements from law firms touting their businesses. Some specialize in automobile, workers' compensation, or medical malpractice. The lawyers in the ads are usually quite specific when they tell the viewers how speaking to an insurance representative or other person can impact their claim. Most ads tell the viewers that if they do speak with someone other than an attorney, it might jeopardize chances of successfully settling their claim. The lawyers are not inventing this just to drum up business. You can be sure that when they say your insurance company or your employer will be consulting with their attorneys, they are not just using this as a ploy to have you call them. You have heard it before, but you need to remember—the insurance carrier will do whatever it takes to limit their financial liability without giving any thought to what it will cost you.

## Be Truthful

If you are someone who might have a problem telling the truth or tends to embellish, you are probably better off saying nothing. Insurance fraud is a very serious offense. Tell the truth, or keep quiet and let your attorney speak for you. Do not discuss the case with your family and friends. If the defense wants to dispute the claim in court, they may be able to call your family and friends as witnesses to support their side of the claim using your own words or actions against you. Do not expect that they will lie for you or perjure themselves and risk their own legal troubles just to protect you.

You must also remember to be truthful with your attorney. If you hire a lawyer to represent you, and you have lied about your condition or certain specifics of your claim, you may be discredited and the lawyer may request that you find another attorney. If your deception is not discovered until you are in a legal proceeding such as a deposition—or worse, at a hearing—you risk a dismissal or the loss of your claim.

You should also expect your lawyer will be honest with you. When you set up your client-attorney relationship, you should ask how you will be kept up-to-date on the status of your claim. You should ask very specifically if your attorney will meet with you occasionally, send you a letter of update or copy you on all correspondence. You are a consumer of the legal services offered by your attorney. You have a right to know how things are going and what the plan is. If it has been a long time since you heard from your lawyer, give her a call; or better yet, write her a letter and ask what is going on with your claim. It is unlikely that your case was set aside and forgotten, but it is not impossible. If this is the case, it could have a serious impact on the outcome of your legal claim. Remember, you are the consumer. You should always know what you are paying for.

### To Retain An Attorney Or Not

No one will tell you whether or not to retain an attorney. If you have a workers' compensation claim, there are various state regulations which affect an attorney's participation in your claim and how the claim may proceed. There are some things you need to know when trying to decide whether to hire an attorney or not.

Most attorneys can tell you after your first screening call if they feel that they can assist you. You might be asked to come in for an initial consultation with the attorney to review the issues surrounding your claim. If the lawyer feels that she can get a successful outcome of your claim, you will be asked to sign a retainer or statement of representation which confirms your arrangement with the lawyer. Before you sign, it is important to understand the financial obligations of this agreement. State agencies which regulate workers' compensation claims usually have specific laws about the fees that attorneys can charge a workers' compensation claimant. The laws are specific regarding how and when the attorney will collect her fees. In some states, the fees come out of the final permanent partial impairment settlement, or in others, it may come out of your weekly/bi-weekly compensation check. Some states allow for a set fee (for example, 33 1/3%), while others will allow for the inclusion of expenses. Whether your claim is for a workers' compensation, disability or liability claim, it is very important to clarify how much you will pay and when. It is also important that you clarify if there is the possibility of additional costs related to expenses the lawyer might incur while managing your claim. Be sure to ask for a specific list of the kinds of charges which might be considered expenses falling outside the scheduled fees—they might cost a lot more money than you ever expected.

### Claims Other Than Workers' Compensation

Not all workers' compensation claimants will require representation by an attorney. They may have simple, uncomplicated claims for injuries or medical conditions. They may have routine recovery times. They may return to work without any problems. But there are some claims filled with complications from the beginning. If you are not a workers' compensation claimant, but have an injury, illness, complication from a treatment, or a health issue which is the result of another's negligence, you should speak with an attorney. A consultation will help decide if it is worth your time, and the attorney's, to try to pursue another claim. For most other types of liability claims, the attorney is usually hired on a contingency basis. This means that she will take a fee only if you have a successful claim (win your case) against another party. As with workers' compensation claims, your contract may specify that expenses will be added to your final bill from the lawyer. Again, it is important not to overlook this part of your retainer agreement. In most instances these expenses are required to prepare your case or defend your claim. Some attorneys have set fees which they charge for specific types of work. You need to be clear about what your lawyer will cost you.

### The Settlement May Affect Your Other Benefits

If you expect a settlement such as that received in a permanent partial disability disbursement in a workers' compensation claim, it is important that you understand how this may affect other benefits which you may be receiving. For example, if you are a workers' compensation claimant and your state allows for the lump sum distribution of any settlement at the conclusion of your claim, and you also receive Social

Security Disability, it is important that you speak with your attorney or the other agency involved to determine if there is any withholding of which you might be unaware. If you are a Medicaid recipient, it will be important for you to understand how additional monies available to you may impact the social services dollars you receive on a monthly basis. If you receive a settlement amount from workers' compensation, you will need to understand if your Social Security Disability payments or Medicaid benefits will be withheld to make up the difference of the settlement. If you have both a workers' compensation claim and a medical malpractice claim, you will need to know what happens when you receive a settlement from one insurance carrier. For example, if you settle the medical malpractice claim for a large sum of money, you will need to know if the workers' compensation carrier is entitled to the funds that they have paid from that settlement.

## Do You Need A Medicare Set-Aside?

In an effort to reduce costs paid by Medicare and the Social Security Disability Insurance (SSDI) system, the federal government has adopted a series of regulations which can directly affect settlements that people receive, whether they are workers' compensation or liability insurance recipients. The regulations are very complex, but they state that if there is a "reasonable expectation" that a person receives or is likely to receive SSDI benefits in the next thirty (30) months or is a Medicare beneficiary, and the settlement is expected to be more than $250,000.00, a Medicare Set-Aside (MSA) Allocation must be completed prior to a settlement.

Make sure that when you are discussing your settlements, the issues of MSA allocations are discussed and clarified. A MSA can have long-term effects on your financial situation. Do not jump at the first big settlement offer that comes your way. You need to remember there is the possibility that a large portion of your settlement is going to a set-aside trust, and a certain percentage—plus expenses—is going to your attorney. You must now ask the bottom-line question: How much do I actually end up with in my pocket?

An MSA is a projection or Life Care Plan of a person's expected medical costs over their remaining lifetime (life expectancy). For example, an MSA includes physicians visits, possible surgeries, therapies and/or treatments, medical equipment and medications, etc., that a person is expected to use for his medical condition over the remainder of his life expectancy. The MSA is based on past trends of the types of care the patient has received. It also is based on the potential future care that might be expected based on the standards of care to manage his condition.

If the MSA is not completed and the information is not presented to the Centers for Medicare and Medicaid Services (CMS), there is a strong likelihood that any future medical claims will be denied by Medicare/SSDI. These are complex issues you need to discuss with an attorney. The MSA is federally regulated and—in some cases—may not be optional, depending on the specifics of the anticipated settlement. All information regarding settlements goes into national databanks and registries that Medicare can reference to make sure the proper MSA procedures have been followed. As future claims are processed, Medicare can check these registries to make sure that they do not pay out funds for something already earmarked in an MSA account.

If claims are denied, they may be denied without any option to appeal. I have worked with some attorneys who believe that obtaining an MSA is up to the carrier. I have worked with some carriers who believe that obtaining an MSA is up to the plaintiff. In any case, it is advisable for you to ask your attorney about the MSA process. If an MSA was not established and should have been, a person who then has his claims denied by Medicare may need to pursue a legal action against the parties in the claim (the carrier and defense team, and possibly the plaintiff attorney) to have these denied claims covered.

For example, consider the following: If you and your lawyer agree to a settlement amount of $275,000.00, and your future care expenses related to the injury or illness that led to that settlement are expected to be $200,000.00, you may only see $75,000.00 of the settlement in a check to you. It may be even less once your attorney fees are deducted. The rest (the $200,000.00) will be placed in a Medicare

Set-Aside allocation/trust, to be used for your future medical needs. This is in sharp contrast to the past, when a person could receive his full settlement amount and use the funds as he chose. Now the government has put a system in place to reduce some of their costs and shift the burden of those costs back onto the people in the country.

### Legal Malpractice

As you progress with your claim, it is important to maintain open communications with your lawyer to make sure that you understand the status of your claim and your rights under the claim. An attorney can be invaluable in protecting your rights. If you retain an attorney and are having difficulties and feel that your attorney is not working to represent you to the fullest extent of your contract with him, you can call your local or state Bar Association grievance committee to discuss your concerns. Attorneys are bound by very strict codes of ethics. Unlike physicians, if an attorney is found to be in direct violation of the rules of ethics, he may be severely sanctioned, and publicly so. Physicians might have a malpractice case, or be sanctioned by their governing professional conduct board, but the system of sanctions is usually a closed, peer-review system—making it still very difficult to find out the physician's record. Unless a physician has a consecutive series of malpractice complaints, it is unlikely that there will be a public airing of the offense.

### Things To Remember

- Have an initial consultation with an attorney to review your claim.
- Make sure that the attorney specializes in the type of legal matter at hand.
- If you feel that your employer or someone else may be responsible for your illness or injury, an attorney can clarify how to best proceed.
- Medical malpractice may complicate your claim.
- Product liability may complicate your claim.
- The insurance company has their own attorneys; you will be better protected with your own attorney.
- Do not discuss your claim with anyone except your attorney or someone with whom he advises you to discuss the issue.
- Be truthful in your representation of the situation when talking to your attorney.
- Understand the financial agreement you will have with the attorney.
- Clarify the financial agreement and get a specific list of what "other expenses" might include.
- Understand the implications of a settlement on other benefits (such as Medicaid) which you receive.
- Inquire if you will need a Medicare Set-Aside and, if so, what it will mean to the settlement of your claim and distribution of that settlement.

### Questions You Need To Ask

- What can an attorney do for me and my claim?
- How much will it cost for an initial consultation with the attorney?
- How much will it cost to retain an attorney? How and when will the attorney be paid?
- Does the attorney I wish to retain specialize in the type of claim that I have?
- If I am dissatisfied with the services provided (or not provided) by my attorney, what recourse do I have?
- What are the specific charges that my attorney has charged to my account?

- Have I given my attorney an honest accounting of my injury or condition and any past problems which might complicate or reduce my claim?
- Is my attorney providing me with updates on the progress in or obstacles to my claim?
- Do I know with whom I should talk and what I should or should not discuss with others besides my attorney?
- If I am to receive a large settlement will I need to have a Medicare Set-Aside prepared? If the settlement is in the form of a structured settlement, how will that or an MSA affect my access to the funds of the settlement?
- Does having an attorney get me more money and/or benefits than I might otherwise receive?
- How much of the settlement actually ends up in my pocket, after the attorney gets paid and the Medicare Set-Aside is set up?

## *Follow-Up Medical Care And Rehabilitation Options*

When your doctor discharges you from the hospital, it is easy to assume that your care is nearly over and that you are, as they say in baseball, home free. Not so fast. Most illnesses and injuries require at least some post-care—if not complex follow-up—with several doctors, as well as inpatient or outpatient rehabilitation. Your follow-up care can last for weeks, months or even for the rest of your life. Make sure you know what comes next for you.

### Follow-Up Care

Once you have established your claim (if you have a workers' compensation or disability claim) and are working with a physician or other healthcare provider, you will most likely require additional follow-up care and evaluations. Follow-up care can be managed in several ways. The most common follow-up is for you to return to the doctor who initially diagnosed your problem and treated you. Once you are stable or your injury has healed, you are discharged from his care and do not need to come back.

There are a few things to check on before you start going back to see the doctor or other healthcare providers. You should clarify with the carrier if there is a limit to the number of times that you may follow-up with the provider without obtaining a prior certification for additional visits. You should also find out if there are certain physicians who participate with your particular insurance.

### Managed Care Systems

Your state may have rules and regulations which mandate that a workers' compensation or disability claim be coordinated through a formal managed care system. Your non-work-related claim or Medicare/Medicaid may also be part of a managed care system. In either case, if there is to be payment made for your treatment, and you are part of a managed care system, you must follow the guidelines of that system. If your insurance carrier follows a managed care approach, it is most likely that you will only be allowed to see a certain group of providers and physicians who are part of their system. Each state has different rules about this. You should find out what your state agency says about your particular situation. This is especially important if you expect that they will pay the doctor or provider fees. You must also clarify what your co-pays and financial responsibilities will be if this is not a work-related claim.

### Out-Of-Network Providers

Do not assume that just because you have a work-related injury or illness that you have the right to see providers wherever and whenever you choose. Additionally, if your illness or injury is being handled by private insurance, there may also be limits on *whom* you can see. The insurance company paying the bills makes the rules. If you want to see a physician or provider outside a given network, you may be required to pay out of your own pocket for the service. If this is a workers' compensation claim, you may be allowed to change providers after a certain period of time. You may also be limited as to the number of changes you may make. For example, if you find a doctor you would like to start seeing, make sure that she is part of the referral network for whichever insurance you have. You will need to check with your carrier or state agency about this. This is especially true for workers' compensation. You may be restricted to a certain list of doctors even though you found one who you think will help you the most. Most providers are aware of the restrictions regarding the need to comply with the state's rules and regulations.

If you have seen a doctor whom you like and later were told that you cannot continue to see her, you can probably file an appeal to at least have the existing charges covered. If you trust this doctor and feel that she is completely on your side, and you will not be allowed to return there under your current coverage, ask her if she has the name of someone she trusts to whom she can refer you. There are some carriers who will put up a fight if you want to make this change. If that is the case, check with your lawyer or call the state agency to see how you can see the doctor of your choice.

If you are in a managed care or disability system, you *may* have the option to pay for part of the services if they are not covered. If you are part of the workers' compensation system, you may not have that option. However, never take your adjustor's word about this, clarify it with a regulator. A regulator is a person who works for the agency or state department overseeing the workers' compensation system in your state. Go to your state's workers' compensation homepage on the Internet or ask your employer to obtain the phone number of this agency. I have been told by several state agency representatives (when calling to clarify benefit information for clients) that adjustors will say anything to keep costs down, even if it is not true.

## Precertification

Precertification is the same as prior authorization. It simply means that something—whether it is a doctor appointment, surgery, physical therapy, etc.—has been approved prior to your attending the appointment. It is important to know both if a specific appointment and a certain number of visits have been precertified, and for how long that certification is valid. Oftentimes, when a patient goes for treatments such as physical therapy, there will be a certain number of visits approved at a time. These visits are expected to be used within a relatively short period. For example, twelve visits may be approved for a two-month period of time. If additional treatment is needed, a recertification can usually be obtained, especially if there is documentation of medical necessity. Recertification means that the original precertification or prior authorization has been extended. If you continue to improve, additional treatments or visits will usually be authorized.

## Additional Treatments

If there is a request for additional treatment, this request is usually accompanied by either a phone call and/or written medical reports that will detail your progress to that date. If the carrier believes additional therapy is considered maintenance therapy (therapy intended to help you keep the level of improvement and function already achieved from your rehabilitation), it may be more difficult to get the additional treatments authorized. Let's assume that the documentation indicates that you are nearing maximum medical improvement (MMI) or medical end result (MER; the point in your recovery at which you are not expected to make any additional gains), it is likely that a recertification will be either denied, or approved for only a few more treatments or visits to the physician.

Many insurance companies—including Medicare, Medicaid and the managed care companies—set limits on the number of times a certain treatment can be provided. For example, some companies may limit chiropractic care to a certain number of treatments per year. The companies may also require ongoing documentation of proof that you are continuing to improve. If additional treatments are denied, and your provider (doctor, physical therapist, chiropractor, etc.) thinks you would benefit from additional care, you may have to provide this sort of documentation before any additional care is approved. If you have been denied, make sure that you understand what you need to do to continue your care. If you continue to see the provider and receive care that has not been approved, you might be stuck with the bills. Always keep in mind that you can usually appeal a denial, but be sure that you and your providers are working on the same page, and your appeal efforts are supported.

## A New Physician May Be Beneficial

If you have a physician state that you are at MMI but a review of your records and progress suggests this is not the case, it may be necessary to file a written, urgent appeal to obtain authorization to see a new provider and receive any treatments he prescribes. If you have an attorney, she can help you with this appeal. If it is evident to the new physician that there are additional benefits which you would receive from his care, your new physician may decide to begin treatment before his care is authorized.

Some physicians believe that a patient's needs and the benefits the patient would get from timely treatment far outweigh the risk of a denial of their bill. Your best hope is that the new physician can and will support your appeal and obtain a reversal of the denial. However, many physicians and ancillary providers may not be willing to take on this financial risk. It is difficult to talk about reimbursement with your physician. However, it is better to talk about finances and carrier restrictions than to be humiliated when you arrive for a visit and find out the service has been denied. Most physicians are very aware of reimbursement guidelines. They may be doctors, but they are also running a business. If you know that the service has been authorized, but the physician or provider tells you that they have not been paid and are suspending your treatment until payment is received, you need to call the state agency and your carrier immediately—from the provider's office—to clear up the problem. Here is where having your binder with you can be very helpful.

## Getting To The Appointments

Once follow-up care is prescribed or rehabilitation plans are in place, it becomes your responsibility to follow the plan and show up for your appointments. Most insurances require that you arrange for your own transportation to and from appointments. However, there are some carriers (usually the workers' compensation or disability carriers) who recognize that there are individuals who have no one to help with this. They understand that relying on public transportation or paying for private transportation is too much of a burden for the patient. The carrier may recognize it is better to arrange to have you transported—either by a transportation carrier with whom they have previously contracted, or perhaps through a local agency.

Some towns and cities have agencies dedicated to getting people back and forth to their medical appointments. If the carrier understands that you have no way to get to your medical appointments, they may realize that it would be foolish not to provide transportation—especially if not doing so will contribute to a delay in your recovery. States may or may not have specific rules about this, but first check with the insurance company or the state agency to clarify your options. You can also call your local Medicaid or outreach agency to see what is available in your region. If you drive yourself or your family drives you, keep track of the mileage. A Mileage Log is provided in Appendix B.

## If You Are Not Improving

Once treatment is prescribed and you are going to your follow-up appointments as scheduled, it will still be necessary for you to know what is going on with your care and progress. If you feel that something is not right, or you are getting worse instead of better, or if you feel that the treatment is not taking care of your condition, it is up to you to say something. Speak up and request that a reassessment be completed to determine if the current plan is the best for you. For example, if you are getting worse instead of better, notify your doctor immediately. Do not continue to do something if it is worsening your condition. You may have to do some research to see if what you are experiencing is normal for your situation.

You should speak openly with your provider. Make sure that you get your records and read them. Once you have them, make sure that they accurately reflect your complaints. It is not unusual for you to have a lot of complaints that are never documented. It is also not unusual for a provider to write down that you are progressing satisfactorily when, in fact, you are not. If you feel that you are worsening but your provider states in his records that you are improving, bring this to his attention and make sure the record is corrected. It may be uncomfortable for you to do this, but if you do not it is possible that any future care you need could be compromised by this inaccurate information. Future decisions about MMI status and your benefits may hinge on these records. You were told earlier that the carriers are waiting to receive information which will allow them to reduce or terminate your benefits. You may be sent for an independent medical evaluation (IME) with a doctor the carrier has chosen. The IME physician may use the inaccurate information in conjunction with his exam to form a potentially biased opinion. This assessment could then negatively impact your future care and result in denials for additional services.

If you speak to the provider about inaccurate documentation, be prepared to see it in his reports that you have questioned the records. Most providers will be professional and not attack you personally. However, you might see statements in their records that begin to question your motives.

Walter's physical therapist and doctor were writing reports that indicated he was making progress after his lower back surgery; however, when Walter questioned inaccuracies in the reports and complained bitterly of his poor progress and severe pain, his doctor made a statement questioning Walter's motives. The doctor wrote in the records, "There may be secondary gain issues at play here." This doctor was implying that Walter's complaints were simply a ploy to extend his workers' compensation weekly benefits. Walter was smart enough to request a transfer to another doctor. Some serious complications were discovered on repeat testing. The tests showed there was some damage to the nerves which had not been identified by the previous doctor. Walter was now no longer a candidate for any care that would help his situation, because the damage and scarring of the nerve was permanent and unable to be surgically repaired. Walter's doctors and therapists had not listened to his complaints; as a result, Walter now suffers from a severe, chronic pain syndrome.

If you do some research about your problem, and you can find supporting evidence which confirms your suspicions, bring this to the attention of your physician or provider immediately. If she will not listen to you, find a new provider or doctor. Complaining that care is not working does not mean that you are trying to manipulate or get more money from someone; it means that what is being done to this point is not working and a new plan needs to be made.

On the other hand, you may not have any new problem, and what is happening is expected. You cannot know either way unless you address the question. One of the worst things a patient can do is to sit and stew and worry that there is a problem, and then not ask anyone about it. It may go against your inclinations, but you really need to speak up and address the problem sooner rather than later. If you feel really uncomfortable pointing out the inaccuracy between symptoms of which you have complained and what was written, bring someone with you and have him address the problem for you.

## The Physical "Terrorist"

It cannot be repeated enough: If you feel that you are getting worse instead of better, speak up! There are some providers who strictly adhere to the "no pain, no gain" theory of rehabilitation. This can be appropriate for many patients, but not for all.

Mark had received physical therapy services from several therapists over a couple of years. Mark had a very limited tolerance for any type of discomfort and would complain bitterly if the therapists tried to advance his program. Most of the providers gave in to Mark's smallest complaints of discomfort and did not push his limits. They stopped pushing him forward and lowered their goals. His care ultimately suffered. A re-evaluation with a new surgeon, a final surgery, and a referral to a different therapist who was more knowledgeable about Mark's specific condition were the keys to his recovery. But none of this came without a high cost to Mark; he had become used to controlling the rehabilitation providers in an effort to control any discomfort that developed. Unfortunately, this unconscious control extended his disability by over two years. It caused him to be anxious, distrustful of everyone, and depressed. His self-esteem and self-reliance suffered. His family life suffered. Finally he met the therapist who turned his situation around. Sue, a real hard-nosed individual, became fondly known by Mark as his physical "terrorist." She pushed him to his limits, physically—and then just a bit more. Sue listened when Mark had complaints and referred him back to his doctor to make sure no new problems were developing. When she knew it was safe, she pushed him more. Mark was finally able to become independent and retrain for a new job that fit with his restrictions. He regained his sense of pride.

If you are working with a physical "terrorist" be sure that you are progressing and not *regressing*. Make sure she is listening to you and planning your care based on where you are and not where she thinks you should be. Not all physical therapists who are aggressive and assertive are meeting your individual needs. However, the opposite is also true. If you have a therapist who does not push you hard enough to help you meet your goals, your needs might not be met, and your care may suffer.

### Avoid Wasting Time

If there is a problem in your follow-up care, do not assume that somebody else will identify the problem and take care of it. You need to continue to be your own best support. If you are unable to do this, it will be necessary to have a representative continue to work for you. If you are scheduled to have a referral to a new provider for additional follow-up care or treatment, you will need to do your homework and make sure that this is the appropriate referral for you. There is nothing more frustrating than to be referred to a physician for his assessment, only to have the physician tell you that this was a waste of time and that there is nothing he can do. Each time you have an appointment with a doctor or other healthcare provider who cannot add something to your treatment plan, you waste valuable time. Such delays can prolong your recovery and possibly contribute to future disability.

### Dialogue Is Essential

As you do your research on your injury or illness it will be important to learn about the national standards for your particular problem. You will need to learn of what the current and ongoing treatment should consist. You can find this information by checking out websites, calling a local chapter associated with your disease, or going to the library. If research suggests that a certain type of care is often prescribed, but it has not been prescribed for you, ask your doctor to explain his rationale. All providers are not working off a universal set of standards and algorithms for each diagnosis. Each physician is trained differently; therefore each physician has a different algorithm or treatment protocol which he uses to treat certain diagnoses and complaints. If you feel that your physician is really missing the boat and not following treatment guidelines which are routinely and widely accepted, you should bring this up as soon as possible. If he will not even consider any other options, and cannot—or will not—give you a satisfactory answer as to why, consider changing providers or at least obtaining another opinion. Do not change just because the doctor says no to a recommendation; sometimes there are treatments that are routinely ordered, but may not be appropriate for your specific problem. You will need to clarify if this is the case. There may be a medical reason that explains the discrepancy. This is where open dialogue with your provider is essential to your recovery.

### Inpatient Rehabilitation

If you have a more serious injury or illness, you may also be a candidate for inpatient rehabilitation at a facility specializing in intensive multi-disciplinary rehabilitation. This means that the facility addresses all of your physical, emotional, and occupational care needs. You stay there while they care for you. Some people who require inpatient rehabilitation have suffered from serious injuries or illnesses and are unable to advocate for themselves. They may or may not be more dependent upon their representative to advocate for them. Your condition and the accessibility to the facilities will help determine which facility will be best for you. Most patients who are admitted for inpatient rehabilitation must meet specific criteria before admission.

There are *acute* and *subacute* rehabilitation facilities which provided multi-disciplinary care. In the *acute* inpatient rehabilitation setting, the patient's needs are usually quite complex, requiring skilled care that addresses a multitude of physical and emotional needs. Patients transferred for acute inpatient rehabilitation may be medically stable, but their medical condition is complex and still in flux. These are patients whose care could not be safely managed or coordinated in a home setting with available homecare services.

*Subacute* rehabilitation is appropriate for the patient who requires a more intensive multi-disciplinary program than is available in an outpatient setting. Subacute rehabilitation is usually reserved for the patient who requires several hours of therapies, treatments, and interdisciplinary assessments, which could not reasonably be rendered in the outpatient or home setting. The number of visits required for the care during a day would be too exhausting and difficult to coordinate. At the time of a subacute admission, the patients are usually medically stable. These are patients who—if no subacute bed was available—could safely go home with homecare services.

The rising costs of healthcare have led to more innovative methods of treating patients outside of the hospital setting; however, these patients usually require a level of care which is too skilled and demanding for their families to try to provide. For example, a young motor vehicle accident survivor with multiple fractures may need to become more independent with ambulation and wound care prior to going home. Patients who recently had total joint replacement surgeries are also excellent candidates for subacute rehabilitation. Patients who have had extensive surgery—and are weak and unable to take care of themselves, because they need more strengthening—are candidates for a subacute rehabilitation program. Patients who have flare-ups of chronic illnesses, but have the potential to regain some of their pre-flare-up function, are candidates for the subacute setting. Oftentimes, physicians will plan a post-op transfer to a subacute facility when they are scheduling elective surgery. If you have suffered a serious injury or undergone an extensive surgery you might benefit from additional care before being discharged home to care for yourself. Have a family member or a friend call your physician to discuss the possibility of transfer to a subacute facility.

## Fear Of Going To "The Home"

One issue that frequently comes up during discussions about the subacute transfer process is that many subacute rehabilitation facilities are new extensions of skilled, long-term care facilities (nursing homes). Many older people fear being sent to "The Home." Younger patients are sometimes equally concerned. Many worry about being abandoned with "those old people." Most subacute facilities have adult patients of all ages, from eighteen years old and up. There are also subacute facilities for children and adolescents. Any adult who is considered for subacute rehabilitation will have to meet strict criteria prior to transfer to the facility. One of the main criteria is that the rehabilitation process is expected to be completed within a given amount of time (usually three to four weeks). If a patient requires more complex rehabilitation for a greater period of time, they will most likely be considered for an acute rehabilitation facility which focuses on specific diseases or injuries.

## Before Your Transfer

Prior to transfer to another facility, the hospital and rehabilitation staff will make all of the necessary arrangements for your transfer. They will coordinate the logistics, and negotiate acceptable rates to cover the costs of your stay. If you are a Medicare or Medicaid recipient, the facility will be bound by their respective guidelines. If you will be self-paying, it will be up to you or your representative to clarify the financial issues *before* your transfer. Regardless of your source of payment, it is important that you or your representative be aware of all of the conditions of your transfer.

## Get The Discharge Plan On Admission

When a person transfers to subacute from an acute care facility it is important that the discharge plan start on admission. This reassures the patient that her care has an expected end date, and it allows the family or caregivers to prepare for the eventual return home of the patient—especially if there are ongoing special needs. Throughout the subacute stay, the patient and her representative(s) will get periodic assessments with updates on her progress and treatment plans. The goal for the subacute patient remains focused on discharge.

### The Acute Rehabilitation Patient

For some patients, their illness or injury may be more severe and require even more intensive inpatient rehabilitation. Some of these patients will be able to return home, while others may regain a limited amount of functional ability before they are transferred to a long-term care facility or nursing home. Patients who are admitted for acute rehabilitation typically have more severe, complex injuries or illnesses which require more skilled interventions and assessments than subacute patients.

### You Need An Advocate!

Remember what you learned before: The adjustor who is negotiating with the rehabilitation facility is working for the insurance company. The adjustor is not there to be your advocate. His business is to save money for the carrier. Saving money pays his salary. He will try to limit your rehab stay and get you home as soon as possible. The rehabilitation staff should be working to make sure that you only leave when you are medically safe to leave. The rehabilitation staff should be protecting your interests; however, they also are a business and will be looking to begin or continue their business arrangement with the carrier for future patients (business). If you feel that your care and follow-up are more focused on the insurance company rather than you, get in touch with the agency that regulates workers' compensation or the insurance in your state to find out what your rights are under the law.

Regardless of the course of rehabilitation and follow-up, it is necessary for each patient to have an advocate. If you can assume the role for yourself, this will help you maintain independence and control. If you have an injury or illness which leaves you incapable of handling this role, it is necessary for you to appoint an advocate who can maintain a close relationship with the rehabilitation staff. He can then assure that your treatment and discharge plans meet your needs. As your rehabilitation and follow-up progress to your maximum medical improvement (MMI), it will be necessary for you to remain focused on your needs and goals.

### Another Opinion Counts

A final caution on follow-up care and your rehabilitation: If you get a differing second (or third) opinion from another physician on the treatment that you have received thus far—or on the treatment planned—you should obtain *another* opinion. If this conflicting opinion comes from a physician hired by the insurance company, you should get an opinion from a physician that you hired. Remember, any physician hired by the carrier usually offers an opinion that will save the carrier money, whether or not it is best for you. It can be very confusing to receive a different opinion on how care should progress. If you are confused about additional rehabilitation care, you will need to do some research. You should not be doctor-shopping to find someone who tells you what you want to hear. Getting another opinion is intended to help you sort out questions you may have when you are given conflicting opinions.

The carrier will try to limit the amount of money that they spend on your claim. They may try to stand in the way when you want to get another opinion. The carrier may even try to bully you and threaten you with stopping your benefits if you try to go to another doctor. If you are in the workers' compensation system, some states have very specific laws that tell claimants with whom they can and cannot treat. If the carrier does not approve the physician to whom you go, they might deny the doctor's bill and stop your benefits, saying that you are not following prescribed care. Now is when you will need to launch an appeal, possibly with the backing of an attorney.

Your success on appeal will depend on several things, among them that you have followed all of the legal procedures for the appeal (thus the need for a lawyer). But you will also need to carefully and completely document any benefit that you have obtained since making the change. It may be that the courts will side with you—especially if you can prove that you were getting nowhere with the previous physician, but have now made improvement. If you feel that you have a legitimate concern and you get a denial from the carrier, appeal to your state agency. If your claim is billed under your private insurance, depending on your insurance plan you may also be limited to a certain group of providers with whom your insurance has contracted. This may be especially true if you belong to a managed care plan. In the private health insurance sector and the managed care arena, it may be more difficult to win your appeal to see a physician outside the referral network without having to pay a large portion or all of the bill. You should hire an attorney to intervene on your behalf. No matter how many physicians or healthcare providers you see, always remember to get copies of all of their reports, letters, and recommendations. Once you get the information, review it carefully. It will help you make an informed decision.

## Things To Remember

- Clarify your treatment options.
- Understand your co-pay and financial responsibility.
- Learn about your managed care system and its restrictions.
- Find out which providers you can see.
- You are responsible for keeping your appointments.
- If you need transportation, ask the carrier if they can help.
- If you are not improving, ask for a reassessment or referral to another provider.
- Make sure you progress, not regress.
- Make sure the new referral is appropriate to your condition.
- Check out your rehabilitation options.
- Everyone needs an advocate.
- Clarify any differing opinions.

## Questions You Need To Ask

- What are my treatment options?
- What is the expected outcome of each of the treatment options?
- How many times has the provider performed this procedure, and/or managed this diagnosis? What problems and success has the provider obtained?
- Can/will you refer me to another physician outside of your practice group or provider network for an objective second opinion?
- If I am not improving, why not?
- What should/could be done differently to change my progress?
- If I have a conflicting report, what does it mean?
- What treatments are approved by my insurance carrier?
- For what am I financially responsible?
- When is my next appointment?
- What is expected of me between appointments? Do I have restrictions or treatments to follow? If so, what are they?
- How will I get to my next appointment? Have I set up my transportation far enough in advance if I need assistance?
- Do I have an advocate or someone who will accompany me to my appointment?
- Do my providers, carrier and family know who my advocate is?

## Medications And Special Equipment Needs

**I**t is unusual that you will become sick or injured and not require any medicine and/or medical supplies or equipment. You can save yourself a lot of extra headaches if you follow some simple advice about where and how you can get these, and who can help you do it. One of the biggest obstacles to people getting well is that they fail to get their prescriptions filled, or they do not obtain the equipment or supplies they need.

### Who Pays For What You Need?

If you are suffering from an injury or illness, at some point during the course of treatment you may need prescription medications, disposable medical supplies or durable medical equipment. If yours is a disability or workers' compensation claim, these special needs should be covered by the insurance carrier responsible for your claim; but never assume that they will be. Do not assume anything. Make a call to the carrier to see for what they will and will not pay. If you are participating with Medicare or Medicaid, call the regulating agency to clarify what they will cover and how much you will be responsible to pay. Many commercial insurers will deny payment for medicine, supplies or equipment or require a separate rider to the insurance contract before they cover the bills.

Do not be surprised if the carrier requests additional documentation from your physician supporting the medical necessity for the prescribed items. Medical necessity means that the medications, special equipment or medical supplies are needed specifically for the procedure covered under the current claim. Most doctors are aware that they will need to provide you or your carrier with a written statement explaining why you need what they have prescribed. If an item or request for supplies is denied and you feel that the need is directly related to—or is a result of—your condition, you should file an appeal. Be sure to include a supporting letter from your doctor or other healthcare provider documenting the medical necessity for the items or medications. Even with documentation, some things may still be denied. If it is something which your doctor feels is very important to your recovery, inform him it has been denied and ask him to write a letter helping to fight or appeal the denial. If the request is denied again, you may have to file an appeal with the state regulating agency. Once you begin the appeals process with the carrier—for any reason—you should involve the state agency as well. Find out how they can be involved, and send them copies of any letters of appeal which you send. Your final appeal may end up before an administrative appeals judge or arbitrator. You will need all of the documentation that you can gather to argue your case. If you feel uncomfortable handling this alone, consult with a lawyer.

### Durable Versus Disposable Supplies

Many insurers today have set up preferred provider agreements with various medical supply and pharmacy vendors across the country. When an order is written for a piece of equipment such as a walker, a brace or other non-disposable item, this is referred to as a Durable Medical Equipment (DME) item. If you need supplies to change dressings, or personal care which is above and beyond the usual personal needs, you have the need for disposable items. Medications and the items used to administer them (in the case of intravenous drugs, for example) are typically covered under the pharmacy reimbursement guidelines. When these items are prescribed, you should contact your carrier to obtain the name of the vendor (medical equipment supplier or pharmacy) with whom they contract. If you have a Medical Case Manager, she can assist you. If you need supplies or equipment, find out if you must pay up front and seek reimbursement later, or if the carrier will be billed directly by the vendor. Every carrier has different ways to manage pharmacy and durable and disposable supply reimbursement.

### Prepaid Pharmacy Accounts

When prescriptions are purchased directly from your local pharmacy, the costs might be substantially higher than if purchased through a national pharmacy vendor who has contracted with your insurance company. When you speak to your adjustor, ask to have a prepaid pharmacy account set up for you, especially if you are going to be using medications for a long time. The prepaid account can be set up by the carrier (or your case manager) with an individual, local pharmacy or a national vendor. The carrier will arrange for your prescriptions to be either paid in advance or billed to them once the prescription has been filled. This is not the same as a flexible healthcare spending account like you would have through your place of employment. This is also not a prepaid credit card type of account that you can use at numerous pharmacies.

### Which Pharmacy Is Best?

There is no way to say which pharmacy can provide the best service to meet your individual needs. Before heading to the pharmacy or sending your family to fill your prescriptions, you might want to call the pharmacist to find out how much the prescriptions will cost. If you do not have a prescription plan or pharmacy agreement set up by your carrier, you might be shocked when you get to the register. If the price is very high, you should call other pharmacies in the area to see if they offer better prices.

If you have medications that need to be injected or infused (like an intravenous or chemotherapy solution) you may have to obtain the medicine from an infusion company. Infusion companies have a staff of pharmacists, nurses and technicians who prepare and administer the medications for your home use. Their nurses will usually come to administer the drug and watch for side effects. If they do not have nurses available, you may need to have a local nursing agency send a nurse to help you. Or, you might need medication that can be given to you by your family or friends. If you are going to take care of this yourself or with help from your family, call the infusion company and your pharmacy to compare the costs of the medication. Your Medical Case Manager can help coordinate all of this.

### The Difference Can Be Staggering

The difference in the costs of medications can be staggering, and where you obtain the medicine can play an important role in the costs.

Jess needed to have a low-dose chemotherapy agent on a weekly basis for several years to treat an auto-immune disorder. He did not have a prescription plan to cover the cost of medications. This was not a work-related or disability claim, so his health insurance was the primary payor for the mediation. Jess called the insurance company and was told that a good portion of the cost of the medication would be covered under the major medical portion of the insurance because it was an injectable medication. Jess was responsible for the usual co-pay under the major medical portion of his insurance. The medication was obtained—per direction of the insurance carrier—through a local infusion company. The cost of the medication was over $1,700.00 through this supplier. A nurse in the family was able to do the injections, thereby saving additional nursing fees of about $85.00 per hour per week. Jess was responsible for the out-of-pocket fees of 20%, or about $400.00 every 3 weeks for a total of about $7,000.00 per year.

Jess' insurance coverage changed and the new insurance provided prescription benefits. Jess called his local pharmacy and found out he could obtain the drug through them. The new insurance co-pay was now $5.00 per refill, which is about $85.00 per year! He questioned how that could be, as he had paid such an exorbitant amount before. The pharmacist said that the drug only retailed for about $35.00 per refill. A call to the infusion company questioning their inflated price of the medication revealed that the additional charges were for "administrative costs." Therefore, if you are going to be paying out-of-pocket and can use whichever provider you want, you are urged—if time permits—to do some comparison shopping to find out if cost of the drug varies. The mark-up on drugs can be ridiculous.

### The High Costs Of Medications

If you feel that you have been denied the use of a medication because of the cost, the class of the drug, or because it is new drug on the market, you should be in contact with your physician to have him call the vendor or pharmacy directly. Oftentimes the physician may have a specific reason to prescribe a medication which ordinarily would not be covered, and he may be able to persuade the carrier to cover the costs. Many carriers have developed formularies. Formularies are lists of medications which will be covered by the particular carrier. The medications listed in these formularies are usually the older, less expensive medications rather than the newest generation of drugs. Many formularies also list drugs according to a tier system. This system usually has three tiers: Tier 1 for generic drugs, Tier 2 for preferred brand-name drugs and Tier 3 for non-preferred or any drug not covered under the first two tiers. Each tier gets successively more expensive. If you have a co-pay for your prescriptions, you will pay much less for drugs on the Tier 1 list than you will for those on the Tier 3 list. Generic drugs usually refer to the drug by its chemical or non-brand name. For example, a generic drug would be ibuprofen. The Tier 2 or brand name might be called Advil. A drug in the third tier might be a drug from the class of newer non-steroidal anti-inflammatories that has just been released to the market by the manufacturer. The newer the drug to the market, the more likely it is that the price will be very high and part of the third tier of drugs.

If you are prescribed a medication which is not on the formulary, but your physician thinks that this medication would be the best treatment for you, it is up to your physician to document the medical necessity for the medication. If the carrier will not cover the medication, you may have to pay the up-front costs and pursue reimbursement later on through the appeals process. If the financial burden is too great, you need to speak honestly with your physician about it.

Although they are a small group, there are some physicians who are often influenced by what they receive from the drug companies for prescribing the newer generation of more expensive drugs. This is an unethical practice but one that exists. We do not want to believe that unethical behavior in the forms of expensive trips and gifts can influence the way our physicians practice medicine and prescribe medications, but the truth is that it happens, and it happens at the cost of the people who can least afford it. Therefore, if your doctor prescribes a drug that will not be paid for by the carrier, and you cannot afford to pay out of your own pocket, you will need to ask him to prescribe an alternative drug.

### Starter Packs And Samples

There are some instances when you are discharged from the hospital and you may receive a "starter" or sample pack of your medication. This is intended to get you through the period of time before you can get to the pharmacy to pick up your prescriptions. Samples are also used to see if the medication is something you will tolerate without experiencing adverse effects. Some doctors may also offer samples if you are treating at their office. It is a good idea to ask if your doctor has any samples. Not all offices have samples or starter packs at their disposal, in which case you will need to fill the prescription on the way home.

Waiting to obtain your medications can be a problem. Usually if a medication is prescribed, it should be started that day. You do not always have the luxury to wait for the mail-order pharmacy to deliver the medicine in the next week. If you are forced to wait, let your physician know. This delay could be harmful to your recovery and overall well-being. There may be a way your doctor can obtain enough of the medication while you wait for the prescription to arrive in the mail. Usually getting medications through the mail is reserved until you have been established on the medication. In that case, make sure you have a separate prescription to cover you until your medicine arrives.

## Going To The Pharmacy

If you have just left your doctor's office with a new prescription, you will probably want to get it filled before you go home. As we just discussed, before you leave your doctor's office, ask if they have samples. This can tide you over in case you get to your pharmacy and the drug is out of stock. If you get to the pharmacy, and find out that they are out of the drug, ask them to either return your prescription so you can go somewhere else, or—if you are just too sick to go driving to other pharmacies to see if they have the drug—ask the pharmacy staff if they can help you find a pharmacy with the drug in stock. If you can wait for a day or so to start the medicine, ask the pharmacy to tell you when you should come back to pick up your prescription.

Sometimes pharmacies will have limited supplies of some drugs. For example, in my area the pharmacies have a very difficult time getting Methotrexate with preservative. In our case, the pharmacist checked with all the suppliers and called the prescribing doctor, and we had to have the prescription changed to Methotrexate without preservative and then wait for the pharmacy to obtain it. Our pharmacy was actually able to contact the local hospital and purchase enough of the drug to get us through the week until they could obtain enough to fill our prescription for the month.

Sometimes we will be in the middle of a prescription and still have several refills left, only to find out that our pharmacy cannot refill the prescription when we need it. In that case, the pharmacy will not give our actual paper prescription back to us, but they will forward the prescription to another pharmacy that can refill the drug. If they only have a few days' worth of the prescription, they may offer to do a partial refill until their next shipment arrives. Just make sure you have enough medicine to get you through.

If the prescription is for a narcotic—such as OxyContin or MS Contin—and you need a refill, the pharmacy may try to help you out and forward the prescription. Or, they may call your doctor's office and request that a new prescription be sent, voiding out the rest of your refills with them. As there has been so much abuse with some narcotics, it is more likely that you will have to wait a day or so, or get a new prescription, if availability is an issue. If you have the time, before you go to the pharmacy to get your prescription filled, you should first call to see if the drug is in stock. This can save you a lot of time and aggravation, especially if you are not feeling well.

There are mixed responses as to whether a doctor's office will call in a prescription upon request or not. Some offices require at least 24 or 48 hours notice to call in a refill. Some offices require that you call them in advance and they will prepare a prescription slip for you to pick up. You should clarify your doctor's office procedure about prescriptions. In days gone by, doctors would call in prescriptions without much hesitation; today, the volumes are so high that it takes a lot of their staff time just to keep up with prescriptions.

## What If You Cannot Pay Out Of Pocket?

If you have been prescribed certain equipment or medications and are unable to pay out of pocket and will forego the medicines because of the costs, your doctor needs to know. You should also call the carrier and let them know, as this can slow your recovery, delay your return to work, and increase the overall cost of your claim. As soon as your claim is established with the carrier, you should be in contact with the adjustor to arrange for a pharmacy charge account to be set up to prevent any delays in treatment. If you do have to pay up-front for your medications, make sure to keep the receipts and make copies of them to submit for reimbursement.

## Another Pharmacy Issue

When filling prescriptions at your local pharmacy, make sure to keep a copy of your prescriptions or a summary of your medications with you. The other option is to utilize pharmacy providers who have statewide or national databases that can be accessed by the other pharmacies in the group. This will ensure that if you are away from home and have forgotten your medications, you can go to a pharmacy in the town you are visiting to obtain enough of the needed medications to get you by until you return home, or until someone from home can get your medications to you.

If you go to the emergency room in a strange city after discovering that you do not have the medications that you need, you may not be able to obtain either starter packs or prescriptions to tide you over until you receive your medications. This can be especially true if the medications which you require are narcotics. You can be sure that if you go to the emergency room requesting narcotics that you take routinely for a chronic condition, the personnel will be suspicious of—and deny—your request. I have witnessed this scenario time and again. If you have a chronic condition and need medications, especially narcotics, you must be sure to keep the documentation with you. It is sometimes preferable to obtain a letter from your treating/prescribing physician stating what you take and why. This is especially true if you are traveling. There are many people who are narcotic-seeking who have ruined the ability for many people with legitimate needs to obtain the medications they forgot when they traveled. When you travel, it is a good idea to keep your binder or medical summary with you.

### What The Fee Schedule Means To You

A fee schedule is a prearranged fee that is paid for a certain service. For example, an MRI of the lumbar spine may be billed at $1,200.00 by the provider; however, the insurance company or state program fee schedule might say that it is only to be paid at $795.00. You should not pay for anything that should be covered by the carrier. Most companies adjust the bills, especially for many services or items which are part of their fee schedule. This means that they will reduce the amount of reimbursement which is paid back to you for your out-of-pocket expenses. For hospital, physician and other provider services, each state has an established fee schedule used to pay the bills. The fee schedule is used to reduce the costs to the various insurers in the system. Most commercial insurers have established fee schedules as well. If a carrier has a fee schedule, the doctor or provider is usually aware of this and are willing to accept the assigned fee schedule amount.

Many patients do not mind paying up-front for the treatment and submitting their receipts, but this can be a problem once they realize that what they paid might not be what they get back. If you do not keep meticulous records you may overlook some costs that would otherwise be covered by the carrier. You might find that the full price you paid the pharmacist is not the amount that you will receive for reimbursement. In certain circumstances, the patient may be responsible for the balance between the billed amount and the fee schedule amount. This is usually not the case with the workers' compensation system, but you should clarify this with your state or other regulating agency before you start seeing numerous doctors and other healthcare providers.

### Know Which Vendor To Use

If you need equipment or medical supplies, call your carrier to find out with which vendor (supplier) they have a contract or want you to use. You or a family member may have used an equipment vendor in the past, but it is important to realize that they may not have a vendor agreement with your current carrier. If they do not have an agreement with your carrier and you accept merchandise from them, you could be stuck with the bill. This should not happen if the vendor is calling to verify your coverage; however, sometimes there will be an assumption that it is covered—especially if they have done business with you or your family in the past.

### What To Do With Used Equipment

Once the order and payment is in place for your equipment or medical supplies, it is important to understand the arrangement which has been made. Not only will you need to know who is making the delivery and when it is to arrive, but you need to know what your responsibilities are. You need to know if it is your responsibility to notify the vendor to pick up the equipment when you are done with it, or if the item has been purchased for you. Most vendors will check in periodically—especially if you are in a small town—but others simply shift that burden to the patient. Your prescription for the item may specify the amount of time for which you are to have and use the piece of equipment. If you are no longer using the equipment, call the vendor (if it is a rental item) and have it picked up as soon as possible. Let the carrier know when the item was taken back by the vendor, so that the carrier is not paying for something you no longer have. Or, if you are paying out-of-pocket for the rental, do not keep it and pay any longer than is necessary. If the item was purchased for you, and you no longer use it, there are some agencies locally who may take the equipment and loan it to others who are in need and have no way to pay for it.

When a piece of equipment is picked up, get a receipt from the vendor reflecting when it was returned. This is especially important for larger, more expensive pieces of equipment such as hospital beds, continuous passive motion machines, wheelchairs, etc. There are some types of equipment that might be rented for a short period of time, but if you continue to need it and use it beyond that time, it will usually be purchased for you. This is usually true of items like walkers and TENS (TransElectrical NeuroStimulator) units used to help manage some types of pain. These items have a lower price tag, and a prolonged rental would far exceed the cost of an outright purchase. There are some items that can be prescribed where you might get a partial reimbursement from your insurance, such as walkers, canes, or crutches.

Over-the-counter items, such as carpal tunnel wrist supports, are usually not covered. Occasionally such items may be covered, but you will need to call your individual carrier or Medicare to see what is covered and how much they pay for the item. A lot of durable medical equipment such as walkers, commodes, raised toilet seats, etc., need to be paid for up-front and reimbursed once the receipt is submitted. Again, good recordkeeping will help ensure that you receive the proper reimbursement.

## Medication And Prescription Errors

There is one final issue regarding medications and durable medical equipment of which you should be aware. Anyone who watches the evening news or reads a paper will probably have heard stories about patients who received the wrong medication, either from a pharmacist or hospital staff member. If you fear there is a problem with your medication, and you feel that it was prescribed or dispensed in error, it is crucial that you stop using the medicine and report it immediately. You may find immediate assistance and directions to handle the error by calling your regional poison control or emergency management system if the pharmacy is closed. Ideally, you should go to the emergency room for an evaluation to make sure that you will not suffer any adverse physical side effects. Take the container of medication with you, but do not give it away, as you may need this later on as proof of the error. By going to the emergency room you are making sure that you do not suffer any adverse effects from the medication, but you are also documenting that an error occurred. Some states are beginning to have various reporting mechanisms for this type of problem, and the hospital is usually quite familiar with the process. The National Coordinating Council for Medication Error Reporting and Prevention (NCCMERP) is made up of government and private sector agencies overseeing the problems with prescription medication errors, both in and out of the hospital. Many states have laws that address the problems of medication errors as reportable incidents.

Again, do not give up your bottle of medication if there is an error associated with the prescription. If you have suffered a harmful side effect because of this mistake, you may want to consult with a lawyer to determine what your next action should be. This can be especially important if the problem prolongs your recovery, or worse, has long-lasting, negative, permanent effects on your life. If you find a problem, you should document it and add this to your binder. Record any effects and what has been done to correct the problem. If you go to the emergency room, make sure to obtain a copy of your medical record and add it to your binder. It is also a good idea to have your family or an advocate accompany you to the emergency room. Anyone who goes to the hospital for any care should always have someone else with him. There are too many errors and omissions to assume that quality care, free of mistakes, will always be provided.

## Injuries From Faulty Equipment

If you have a piece of equipment which is being used for your rehabilitation, and you suffer further injury or complications due to the failure of that equipment to work properly, you should speak with an attorney. This is an important point, especially if there is documentation in your medical record that indicates you have new problems or complications as a result of the faulty equipment. Many defense firms who will try to carve out these additional expenses from their claim. If this happens, someone will need to pay the balance. If you have not discussed this with an attorney, you might find yourself carrying the additional financial burden. As with medications, if there is a problem you need to make sure to have as much supporting evidence of the problem as possible. In most cases, if the piece of equipment fails, the vendor will pick it up and replace it if you still need the item.

## Document The Equipment And The Injury

If you have the time, you should make every effort to photograph the piece of equipment, including the serial number or other identifying information, or at least write down all of the information for later reference. If you sustain further injury from the piece of equipment due to improper use or application by one of your treating providers, you will need to document all of the information surrounding this event as well.

### *Things To Remember*

- Call the carrier if you have medical supplies or equipment needs.
- Know which vendor to use.
- Clarify your financial responsibilities for the supplies and equipment.
- Find out if and how you will be reimbursed for supplies for which you pay.
- Inquire about a prepaid or direct-pay pharmacy account.
- Let the physician and carrier know if you will not obtain and use the medication due to the costs.
- If you are traveling you may have trouble filling your prescriptions, especially if they are narcotics for chronic conditions. It might be best to utilize a chain pharmacy provider which can readily provide information regarding the medications which you utilize on a routine basis.
- Know what to do with equipment you no longer need.
- Seek care and document any prescription errors and the injuries or complications they cause.
- Seek care and document any equipment failures or complications caused by and injuries sustained from the equipment.

### *Questions You Need To Ask*

- Where can I get medical supplies and equipment? Which vendor do I need to use?
- Does my carrier have a specific provider for medications and supplies?
- Am I responsible to pay for supplies out-of-pocket and seek reimbursement later?
- Will I be fully reimbursed?
- Do I have the necessary documentation from my physician supporting the need for the medical supplies, equipment and medications?
- What do I do with the equipment when I am done using it?
- What do I do with equipment if it is broken?
- Can the carrier arrange for a prepaid or direct-bill account for my prescription and pharmacy supplies?
- If I cannot afford the medications, do I qualify for a program directly from the drug manufacturer which will allow me to get the drugs?

# 10

## *Independent Medical Evaluations*

**I**f you have a workers' compensation, disability or liability claim, it is very likely that you will have to see the insurance company doctor for an assessment. Most people do not understand how this one evaluation can negatively impact or effectively end their claim. The insurance company doctor visit is in most cases called an Independent Medical Evaluation, or IME for short. Some states use different terms such as Utilization Review (UR) Evaluations or Agreed Medical Evaluations (AME). Some carriers will call them Second Opinion Consultations. Whatever they are called, they can all affect the outcome of your claim. Make sure you read the fine print and understand for what the exam is to be used.

### An IME Is Possible, Even Likely

When a claimant has an injury or illness which is being disputed, or he has been treating for a prolonged period of time, or he is in the process of pursuing a resolution to a third party liability process, it is not uncommon to be scheduled for an Independent Medical Evaluation (IME) or a Defense Medical Examination (DME). If an IME has not been scheduled, it is likely that one will be needed to clarify the status of the claim. Some people will say that they have been seen by the state's doctor, the insurance doctor or the "other side's" doctors. All refer to nearly the same thing: an IME/DME. Most times this evaluation is used to determine what further treatment is needed or not needed, or if the claim should be left open, or if it should be closed.

### The IME Versus The DME

Some carriers and some states use the IME/DME terms interchangeably. For this discussion, the term IME will be used as it relates to the workers' compensation system or disability system. The DME is similar in process, but is often used to refer to the exam ordered by the defense team in a third-party liability claim. Both the IME and DME are legal evaluations in which the client sees a physician, paid for by another party, to offer an opinion about the claimant's condition and its relation to the claim at hand.

### AME Versus The QME And The IME

An AME (Agreed Medical Evaluation) is used in some state's workers' compensation systems. The AME is used to make a final determination about various issues in the case. It is used to expedite determinations in the claim and is usually impartial. The decisions and outcomes of the AME are binding for everyone involved in the claim. This is different than an IME, where the decisions are not always binding. When a person is scheduled for an AME, all involved parties (the carrier and defense team, the client and his attorney) agree to follow the outcomes and recommendations made by the AME physician.

A QME (Qualified Medical Evaluation), on the other hand, can be ordered by either the plaintiff or defense. As such, it is not impartial, and often provides the findings sought by the firm requesting the service. The outcomes of the QME are not binding and can be disputed by an opposing opinion. A QME is similar to an IME. The physician who performs either the QME or IME is usually going to offer an opinion that supports whichever side has arranged for the exam.

## The Summons For The IME

If you have a claim that is ongoing or being disputed, you may receive a very official-looking document which demands that you present for an IME at a specific time and place, to a physician whom you probably do not know. The notification will also be quite specific in telling you that if you do not present for the appointment, your claim or benefits may be in jeopardy. If you have any questions or concerns about presenting for this exam, call and get clarification as soon as possible. Do not ignore the notice.

If you are a disability or workers' compensation claimant, or if you are involved in litigation, your state regulations may be quite specific about the IME. The state may specify which physicians are allowed to perform IMEs, what they may charge to perform the test, and what can be addressed in the exam. The state may specify under which circumstances and passage of time relating to the claim an IME can be requested. They may also specify what consequences will be imposed for failure to show up for the IME. If you have a disability or workers' compensation claim, your claim may be closed if you miss your appointment. If you are involved in litigation, it may affect the outcome of your case. If you wish to have someone accompany you to the IME, address this with the party setting up the IME and the physician who will conduct it. If you are notified that you must present for an IME and feel uncomfortable about the process, or have questions or concerns about the physician who is to perform the IME, speak with your attorney.

## If You Cannot Attend The IME Appointment

If there is an exceptional reason preventing you from going to the IME, you will need to notify the carrier (or whomever made the arrangements) well in advance. There are emergencies that arise, but these are rare and will probably be investigated thoroughly if you fail to show up. If you have a problem with transportation and have no way to get to the appointment, you should notify the requestor of the IME immediately. If they want you to go to the IME, they will usually coordinate transportation—at their cost—to make sure that you are able to keep the appointment. If your notification letter says that you must bring certain documents or films with you, do not forget to follow these instructions. The carrier who sets up the exam will most likely forward all of your medical records to the IME physician for review prior to your arrival. It is not uncommon that you will be required to hand-carry all of your films. If transportation to the various radiology providers is an issue and you are unable to get your films, it will be your responsibility to let someone know ahead of time so that alternate arrangements can be made.

## The IME Questionnaire

There are some providers who specialize in IMEs. Some are very thorough and organized and will send you a packet well in advance of your appointment. You may expect the packet to contain a confirmation of your appointment, directions to the facility and how to contact the facility for questions or problems. You might also find a detailed questionnaire that you will be expected to complete prior to your appointment. Many of these questionnaires are lengthy and delve into some very personal aspects of your life. This is going to be part of your legal record related to your claim; be honest when completing the forms. If you refuse to answer parts of the questionnaire—whether at the direction of your attorney, or because you feel that they are too personal—you may see the omission noted in the final IME report. These questions, although quite personal in nature, can help the IME physician to evaluate the extent of your problem. They can also clearly show what impact the injury or illness has on your entire life. If you complete one of these questionnaires, do not forget to keep a copy for your binder.

## Your Advocate At The IME Exam

When you arrive for the IME, you may or may not be allowed to have someone accompany you into the exam room. If it is allowed, your representative may be forbidden to speak, ask questions or generally help you answer questions during the exam, unless specifically queried by the physician. You and your representative may or may not be allowed to take notes or to record the exam. If the IME physician feels that you or the person with you is interfering at all with the exam, the exam may be terminated immediately. If your advocate feels that the DME/IME physician is inappropriate, she can refuse to allow the exam to proceed further. In either instance, this aborted exam can pose a problem for the claimant (you) and should be discussed as soon as possible with your attorney.

## The IME Physician

The doctor performing these exams is not intended to provide or prescribe treatment. He will probably explain this at the beginning of the exam. He is a physician contracted by the insurance carrier, or the defense or plaintiff team, to provide a thorough evaluation of your specific condition as it relates to your current claim. He may also explain that there is no patient/physician privilege as all information obtained during the exam will be provided to the carrier, or whoever set up the exam. This does not mean that you should expect anything less than professional, courteous treatment; it simply means that this is not a traditional patient-doctor exam. When we go to our physicians, we can expect that the privacy of what we say and do is protected under the patient-doctor relationship. This is not the case with the IME/DME physician. He is there to provide an exam and give an opinion on the findings of his evaluation and its relationship to your current claim. He will document anything and everything that is observed during the time of your visit. There will be notes as to how you responded physically to the exam, how you dressed or undressed yourself and how you moved around the office during the exam. He may even document what is observed as you leave the office and walk out and get into your car.

Reports can be so detailed that they include opinions as to whether the physician believed that the patient was faking or embellishing their complaints during the exam. The physician may be so bold as to make a statement which indicates that your reports of discomfort or disability were exaggerated and indicate that the only reason you are complaining is that there are secondary gain issues or functional overlay issues. A statement about secondary gain issues can indicate that the patient is making complaints to get more money or continue their claim. A statement about functional overlay may indicate that there is a mental/psychological reason for the complaints. A physician may use many different phrases to indicate that a patient is faking her complaint. The doctor might suggest that the patient is malingering and does not have a true medical problem. This can be especially true if the tests that have been done (for example, an MRI, x-rays, CT scans, lab work, etc.) are all negative. This does not mean that the patient does not have a real problem, but it does mean that the source of the problem has yet to be identified. However, there are some physicians who do IMEs routinely, or who are biased against certain groups of people or those with certain diagnoses, and even with positive empirical findings, these physicians might still downplay or insinuate that there was some underlying, deceptive cause for the complaints.

## The IME Report

The IME report is not confidential, is shared with all the members of your healthcare team, and may be open to the regulating agency that manages the workers' compensation system. It may eventually show up in the transcript of your court hearing, should you have one. It might even be referenced in a report online and accessed through the compensation system where it is managed. The IME report is confidential as far the confidentiality of medical records is indicated; for example, your exam will not be the topic of discussion for the physician or his staff at their next social function. You will most likely have to contact the carrier directly to obtain a copy of the report. You are entitled to a copy of this report according to your state's Open Records Act. You should make your request for a copy of the IME report via both a phone call and a written request to the carrier. As with all other records, you are strongly advised to read this report in its entirety. If you do not understand it, have your lawyer or a professional help you with the interpretation of the report. There are some IME reports that are so far off-base that they do not begin to accurately provide an assessment of the claimant.

## Disputing The Outcome Of The IME

Most IME reports are complete and address the issues, but many will exclude some very important details. If you find something in the IME report with which you disagree, you or your attorney should formally dispute the report. This should be done in writing. The dispute should then be sent via certified mail to the carrier, the physician who performed the IME, the state agency overseeing your claim, and—if it is an especially glaring issue, which is unprofessional or unethical—also address the issue with your state's agency responsible for regulating physician practices and ethical behavior. You will need to be very specific in this letter of dispute. If you have copies of records, or opinions from your treating physicians which directly contradict the report, you will need to enclose these and reference them to support your argument. You may need to seek your own IME or unbiased second opinion to dispute the original IME.

## Errors In The IME

If you are not sure what the IME report means, you should have someone help you interpret the report. If the carrier or defense attorney paid for the report, they will have little to gain by helping you understand or dispute the report. If you feel there are errors, have an attorney assist you with the dispute if you feel that you cannot effectively manage this on your own. To provide a successful argument to dispute the IME you may need to pay out of your own pocket to have another assessment. This may be especially important if the IME/DME provider will testify to his findings and effectively close your claim. If you have your own assessment done at or very near the same time, you should be able to have your provider testify on your behalf should the dispute progress that far. Make sure to obtain the written report from your physician as soon as possible to support your claims.

## The IME Examination

The physician performing the IME will usually examine only the body part(s) affected by the injury or illness. If the exam causes undue physical discomfort, or if you feel that the examiner is inappropriate in any way, you have a right to verbalize your concern and request that the examiner stop whatever he is doing. It is recommended that you at least have someone accompany you to the exam and wait in the waiting room during your examination. Not everyone feels comfortable with having another person in the room during the exam; however, if you feel comfortable, this may be your best protection in disputing any issues. A first-hand witness is much better for you than someone who was not actually present. A witness may not have the chance to offer a supporting opinion if her witness to the event was from your report only (this falls under the category of hearsay and usually is not admissible in court). You will need to decide what makes you most comfortable, and also consider what you have been directed by your lawyer and personal physician to do.

## Avoid Needless Chatter

Unless you feel you have something significant to contribute to the outcome of the exam, you are strongly advised to avoid any needless chatter and conversation. Politely respond when you are addressed and follow the directions of the examiner, but do not get carried away with offering an elaborate story. Remember that everything you say and do is being observed and will potentially be reported. You can hope that the exam will be an objective evaluation, but do not forget who is paying this physician's bill. There are many physicians who are respectable and very professional, but—like anything else—there are those who will not meet the standards you expect. This is not your personal physician and whatever you say may be twisted and turned around and misinterpreted, or misrepresented, and used to support a negative report.

## The Appropriate IME Specialist

If this is a workers' compensation, disability or other liability claim, this IME can have a significant negative or positive effect on your claim. If you are like most people, you may not understand or appreciate the importance or role that the various certifications in medical specialties can offer to your IME. The various specialty certifications in medicine are too numerous to count. But you should be aware of what the IME practitioner's specialty is. If you have a complicated low back injury, or other neurological condition, you would not want to have an IME done by a physician who is a urologist. This has been done, and sometimes with disastrous results to the claimant's case. Some physicians retire and hope to pick up extra income by offering IME services to the carriers, the state and even the Social Security Administration for their qualifying exams. It is more common that an orthopedic IME will evaluate for an orthopedic problem. Granted, all medical doctors have the same or similar basic medical training, but if it were true that they could treat everything there would be no need for the numerous specialties that currently exist. A basic head-to-toe physical assessment may be the same regardless of the practitioner, but there may be many subtle findings that only a specialist would identify in his assessment. This may be a disputable issue if the report reflects negatively on your overall claim.

## Physiatry And Occupational Medicine Specialists

As with the rest of the medical field, there are physicians who offer IMEs and provide a more specific management for the injured or ill person. It is not uncommon if you have a work-related injury or ongoing disability for you to be referred to a physiatrist or occupational medicine specialist.

A physiatrist is a physician specializing in physical medicine and rehabilitation. Physiatry is a discipline that focuses on the rehabilitation of individuals as they recover from their injury or illness. They are trained in all areas of injury and illness. Physiatrists often work in rehabilitation facilities, or offer their services as Occupational Medicine physicians. Some specialists in this field have extensive backgrounds, training and certifications and are excellent providers dedicated to the successful rehabilitation of their patients.

Some physiatrists or occupational medicine specialists feel that most ongoing or chronic issues can be addressed conservatively. This means that they might recommend more vigorous rehabilitation and non-surgical alternative treatment options, even if such measures have been tried and failed in the past.

## During The IME

During your actual examination you may experience some discomfort or stiffness as the examiner manipulates and examines the affected area. If you feel that the maneuver or exam is causing additional harm or injury, or pain which is intolerable, request that the examiner stop immediately. It is your responsibility to let him know what you are feeling. If you have pain you must let the physician know. Physicians do not read minds. On the other hand, do not embellish. Do not offer a false assessment. Physicians are trained to know what a normal exam should feel like. They may even be able to assess if your complaint is consistent with the physical exam. If the physician asks you to perform a certain activity or maneuver and you feel that you are absolutely unable to do this, it is up to you to say so; but also, it is up to you to explain why you cannot do what he asks. If you cannot move in a particular manner you need to let him know why and what happens when you try this. If you simply refuse without either making the attempt or explaining what your problem is, he may simply report that you were not cooperative with the exam. Even if you explain that you are incapable of a certain maneuver, he may still ask you to try. You should at least make the effort, even if you are unable. Do not force yourself beyond your ability, but make the attempt if at all possible. Sometimes the physician will ask you to try to push a little bit more. If you are able to do so, that is great. If you cannot, then at least he can see that you have tried to cooperate with the exam.

## Reporting Pain In An IME

Pain is a subjective response; it is different for every single person. We have words to describe generally what pain feels like, but to each person, every word can have a different interpretation. Most physicians will respect your complaint of pain or your description of what you feel. On the other hand, if you are with a physician who brazenly states that there is no way your complaint can be as bad as you describe, you are on a slippery downward slope. Do not get sucked into this manipulation. Perhaps for someone else the particular pain would not be described as intolerable, but for you it may be excruciating. Pain at any degree is whatever you say and feel that it is. A simple way to look at the subjective nature of pain is to look at how it affects everyone. For example, there are some women who birth children without the need for any medication or other intervention, whereas there are other women who would request a general anesthetic if they could. No way is better and no complaint is better or worse. If the physician should argue with you about your pain, respectfully request that he accept what you have reported as your best response. If he persists, make a note about the interchange and address this with the carrier in a letter. An ethical physician will never belittle your complaint.

### Document The Events Of Your IME

When you leave the IME appointment, treat this like all of your other provider visits. Make a notation of what happened. This is especially important if you feel that the physician is going to offer a biased account of your exam based on his assessment. As with your other providers, do not wait until you arrive home to make your notes. If you wait until you get home, or for several weeks until you obtain the IME report, your memory may have faded and it may be difficult to relate the exact events of your exam.

### Be Honest During The IME

One last reminder regarding an IME: Be honest and forthcoming with your information. Do not elaborate, but on the other hand do not be belligerent or non-communicative. For example, Carol was very angry and resentful of the entire process. She was rude and would not follow any requests made by the physician. She would not even make an attempt to say "hello." The IME report indicated that she did not have a problem and the current complaints were unfounded. Carol's claim was denied based on that assessment. Unfortunately, she continued to have ongoing problems, but due to her antagonistic attitude, she was not successful in fighting for her claim. It seems condescending to tell adults to be polite, but the bottom line is that it is in your best interest to be pleasant and comply with the exam as best you can, particularly if you end up in a dispute over your claim. If the physician is rude and unprofessional, politely address this and leave the exam. Call the carrier immediately and file a complaint with the state's board for professional conduct issues.

### *Things To Remember*

- You may be required to present for an Independent Medical Exam.
- Failure to show up for the IME can jeopardize your claim.
- Make sure that you bring the appropriate, required documents with you.
- Be sure to complete the questionnaire if one is sent prior to the exam.
- Your advocate or representative, if allowed to accompany you, could jeopardize the IME proceeding if care is not taken.
- The IME physician is not your treating physician and cannot prescribe medications or treatments for you.
- The IME report is owned by the requestor of the exam.
- Request in writing to obtain a copy of your IME report.
- If the IME report is inaccurate, dispute it immediately.
- Avoid needless chatter during the exam. Answer only those questions asked and do not offer information which is not directly solicited.
- Make sure that the IME physician is a specialist in the field pertaining to your injury or illness.
- Follow the instructions of the IME physician.
- Report your symptoms accurately and without embellishment.

- If the IME physician is hurting you, state that there is a problem.
- Make a summary of your IME exam and add to your binder.

## Questions You Need To Ask

- What is an IME?
- Who will pay for my IME?
- What happens to my claim after the IME report is filed?
- How can I obtain a copy of the IME report?
- What will happen to my claim if I fail to present for the IME?
- What can I do if the IME provider is unprofessional and/or seems not to address my specific, individual complaints?
- How can I dispute the outcome of the IME report if it is inaccurate or I disagree with the physician's report?
- How can I arrange for another opinion?
- What is the IME physician's field of practice, and is it appropriate to my problem?
- May I bring someone (my advocate) with me to the IME?
- What if I need assistance in getting to the IME? How can it be arranged?
- Why do I have to arrange to bring records and films to the IME if the insurance company is making me go for the assessment? What happens if I do not bring them?
- What information must I provide at the IME, and what information should I not volunteer because it might be detrimental to my case?

# 11

## Medical Case Management

$O$ccasionally an injury or illness can be complicated and expensive, or fall into a diagnosis category that is known to be a problem for carriers. In an attempt to control the claim, carriers will assign a professional to help coordinate your care in the most efficient and least expensive manner. These professionals are usually called Medical Case Managers or Nurse Case Managers. They should be able to help you and your claim, but remember—they are usually hired by the carriers.

### Medical Case Management Can Be Important

Medical Case Managers (MCM) or Nurse Case Managers can play an important role in coordinating your healthcare. They can be especially helpful to a person with a complex illness or injury. These managers are used most often by workers' compensation carriers and liability insurers in attempts to reduce the high costs associated with ongoing medical care. An MCM is familiar with the medical and rehabilitation resources in your community. As a former MCM, I can address the positive benefits for the patient of working with a Medical Case Manager. As a former Utilization Review Manager for a Managed Care company, I can talk about the benefits obtained by the insurance industry. And, as a former patient who has had two significant injuries to the spine, I can explain both the benefits and the pitfalls of medical case management from the patient point of view.

### What Is A Medical Case Manager?

A Medical Case Manager is usually a registered nurse (RN) who coordinates the medical care you receive. She can oftentimes facilitate appointments and care with various providers and physicians in a timely manner. Historically, because of their medical training and work experiences, nurses make excellent MCMs. They are aware of current medical theories and practices. They understand the multi-faceted complexities associated with recovery and rehabilitation from illnesses and injuries. Nurses are trained to see the whole person and not just the affected body part. The Nurse Medical Case Manager can see how the illness and injury affects the whole person, their family, friends and work relationships. The nurse is trained to work within a treatment plan, coordinating and implementing this plan; assessing and evaluating the patient responses to the treatment plan, and readjusting and intervening again as necessary; coordinating a new or amended plan. A nurse who works as a Medical Case Manager can be most effective in coordinating your medical care needs because she has been trained to be multi-faceted.

Medical case management can be provided in a variety of ways. Medical case managers can work on site, telephonically, or in-house for the carriers. Most MCMs are registered nurses; however, there are some companies who hire vocational case managers to work as medical case managers. Sometimes physical or occupational therapists work as MCMs. A vocational case manager, acting as an MCM, can relay and summarize information, but he is usually not trained or licensed to provide medical assessments, nor does he understand the interactions of procedures, medications, tests, etc. The MCM should be able to understand what it means when a doctor provides a treatment plan or prescribes a medication. He should be able to anticipate the physical response and observe for complications. The MCM should be able to provide you and your physician with any pertinent medical information which he may have observed in his assessments and conversations and meetings with you. He may also have additional information about a medical condition that might impact the current treatment plan, which your doctor either forgot or did not know about. The MCM should be familiar with the standards of care used for various diseases and injuries.

**Field Versus Telephonic Case Management**

Most MCMs work "in the field." This means they work on-site and travel to meet with their clients (patients). The MCM will usually meet with you at your scheduled doctor appointments. She may also meet with you at some of your other healthcare appointments. By being on-site, the MCM can see and hear what is happening in your care, rather than relying on a second-hand report from you or your doctor. She will speak with you and usually your doctor and/or his staff to obtain the necessary information and help coordinate your care. Some MCMs will actually accompany you during your exam. If you feel uncomfortable with the MCM in the exam room while your doctor is checking you over, say so; she can wait and come in after your exam.

The MCM can provide the carrier with a current account of your healthcare status and treatment plans, and update them on your most recent doctor visit outcomes. Some states have mandatory requirements for participation with MCMs. You need to check with your state workers' compensation department to see if it is mandatory that an MCM goes to your appointments with you. If you live in a state that does not require participation with an MCM, you can politely decline to have one accompany you. However, she may still go to the office at the same time you are there to speak with the doctor after your appointment. Some doctors will not meet with MCMs and communicate only by sending written updates of your progress and treatment plans. Sometimes the MCM will appear very sincere and make you feel that your best interests are only what matters, but remember who is paying for her services. She is there to hold costs down and resolve the issues in your claim and get you back to work as soon as possible. If you are not going back to work, she will aggressively pursue documentation from your physician regarding maximum medical improvement.

Remember, you must be cautious about the information you share with an MCM. Seemingly innocent comments and information could be turned around and used against you. Some people would advise you not to communicate with the MCM at all unless you must, such as when the law in your state mandates your cooperation with case management. However, the MCM *can* be an asset to your overall care, especially when she can act as an objective outsider who is not a direct provider of treatment. She can help identify substandard care or offer alternative suggestions for care that have not been considered or provided to you. Do not assume from reading this that you should avoid communication with the MCM, but do remember to be careful about what you say and avoid needless chatter.

There are some nurses who do most of their work with clients via the telephone. They are called Telephonic Case Managers (TCM). The TCM will often hire an MCM to meet with you at some or all of your doctor appointments. The TCM usually has to rely on paper work and conversations with you and the doctor's office staff before she gets the doctor's report. This is especially true if she does not want to wait the several weeks it may take for the doctor's report to reach her. The TCM coordinates care from a distance, possibly even from another state. An efficient telephonic nurse who keeps on top of the information and communication can be just as effective in helping to coordinate your care as a nurse who you see every couple of weeks, or at each doctor visit.

**Pluses And Minuses**

Having an MCM at an appointment with you and your doctor can help the carrier have early access to your updated status. When the carrier knows what is planned, they can approve or deny additional care or benefits without the delays of waiting for written reports. Having an MCM at your appointment can help you get the information you need to understand the doctor's plan. The MCM can explain what the doctor said if you did not understand or cannot remember. This can help you move on to the next step of your care. Waiting for a doctor's report can slow down your treatment plans and progress. If the carrier knows that you need to have surgery or some other tests, they can give the MCM the approval and it can be scheduled without waiting for the paperwork. Sometimes it can take weeks or much longer for doctor reports to reach the carrier.

Having information sooner can also be negative for some patients, especially those who are hoping for another week or two of workers' compensation or disability benefits. If the MCM reports to the carrier that you have reached a MER (medical end result) or MMI (maximum medical improvement) based on her conversation with your doctor, the carrier may begin the process to terminate your benefits sooner than later. After all, their goal is to reduce the money either spent on you or paid to you. An MCM is supposed to provide truthful, accurate reports to the carriers. She is bound by the same ethical standards as any nurse is; however, you must remember who hired her.

### Occupational Health Nurses

There are some employers who keep occupational health nurses on-site. Some states regulate the role of an employer-hired MCM. You will have to check with your individual state about this. Some states limit the amount of direct medical case management that an employee can provide to another employee. Some states believe that there is a direct conflict of interest and will restrict the practice of the Occupational Health Nurse. Some employers use the Occupational Health Nurse as the liaison between the insurance and the human resources department. They also use them to provide immediate emergency and on-site health care for the employees.

There are MCMs who work for national vendors, and there are MCMs who contract independently with various carriers. For the purposes of this chapter I have chosen to separate the nurse's role as a Medical Case Manager from that of a nurse who works in a dual role as both a nurse and a Vocational Case Manager. Some insurance carriers have internal case managers who work collaboratively in the office with the claims managers. It is important for you to know the relationships involved with the assignment of your MCM, as this can impact the relationship that will be developed with you and your healthcare team members.

### Nurses Facilitate Communication

Nurses know the medical language or jargon (as it is sometimes called). They can speak to the physicians and healthcare providers who are part of your healthcare team. By knowing the jargon, they are then able to translate the information into a language that you can understand. It is a given that doctors, by their very nature, are usually rushed and hurried; even their jargon and abbreviations are intended to help them be quick when they write their reports and prescriptions. This might not be such a bad thing, except that this can be very frustrating and confusing to many patients. The average person is usually intimidated by the doctor's hurried manner and strange terminology, and therefore hesitates to push for a clearer picture of what he is trying to say. I have heard time and again, "I don't want to bother him with all my questions." If this is something that you might say, or have said, you need to change that immediately! You are not a bother. This goes back to the issue of informed consent which we discussed earlier. You have every right to be informed; and you cannot expect to be informed if you do not understand the words that are used.

### Never Leave With Unanswered Questions

The MCM can prove a valuable member of your team by helping to make sure that you completely understand your treatment plan and what the physician expects. If you have the chance to meet with your case manager before you go in to see the doctor, you should be able to discuss your questions and concerns. A good case manager should understand and be able to help you make a list of your questions. If you have a personal issue with the MCM assigned to your case, in most instances you can request another MCM be assigned. Usually the carriers will recognize that the outcomes they hope to achieve with an MCM will not happen if you feel uncomfortable with her. One thing to keep in mind is that if you live in a more rural area with limited resources, it is likely that there are a limited number of

MCMs available. You might get a new MCM from the same case management company, which can be frustrating. On the other hand, if you live in a larger area, a frank discussion with your carrier might help you get a new MCM who works for another agency.

The MCM will usually meet with you and the doctor once your exam is completed. This is often a good time to have any questions answered, and to make sure all problems are straightened out before you leave the office. You should never leave an appointment with unanswered questions. If you feel too intimidated or embarrassed to ask certain questions or report certain symptoms, your case manager can be there to support and assist you with the issues. It is also a good idea for you to have your own advocate with you during that meeting with the case manager and your doctor. The majority of physicians will give you as much time as you need to make sure that you understand the issues. But, there are some who rigidly adhere to a predetermined time allotment for each patient they see. They hurry out of the room, leaving many patients feeling rushed, confused and oftentimes neglected and feeling like their problems are unimportant.

## Everyone Needs The Same Information

A trait of a good case manager is the ability to facilitate communication between all of the parties involved with your illness or injury. When you are ill or injured, you become the central figure in the picture. Your physicians, therapists, employer, insurance carrier, attorney, and even your family and friends revolve around you, your needs and your responses to your condition. A good way to picture it is to see yourself as the center of the solar system and the other team members are the planets revolving around you. If you are not the central figure, there is no team and no reason for the other players to interact. A good case manager keeps everyone playing on the same level surface. The MCM's goal is to ensure that you receive the care you need in a timely, cost-efficient, professional and safe manner. The MCM should make sure that all members of the team—including you, the central figure—have the same information regarding diagnosis, treatment plan and expected prognosis. Your rehabilitation cannot be completely successful if everyone involved in your care does not know what the other members of the team are doing. To be successful, each team member must be aware of the others' findings, plans and goals. If anyone, including the patient, withholds information from the other members of the team, your overall recovery and the success of your claim may be jeopardized.

## The Downside

By now you can see that there are many benefits to working with an MCM. But there are potential issues of which you should be aware. There are some medical case management companies who market their nurse case manager services to insurers as money savers. They contract with insurers (carriers) with the sole purpose of saving money for the carrier. These companies keep statistical data which they present in their marketing packages. These statistics are presented in the form of cost/savings analyses.

To satisfy the needs of the carriers and save money, some MCMs will rush care and push for denials of care. The MCM will strive to provide key information that may lead to early releases back to work or denials for future care and benefits. The price to you may be very high. Some case managers will be very conscientious and ensure that the release is safe and appropriate, working closely with the physician to be certain there is no new injury or further complications. Others simply meet the return-to-work or denial-of-service quotas marketed by their employers.

## The Case Manager Is Not Your Friend

If you are a workers' compensation recipient or disability beneficiary whose MCM works for a company with an aggressive return-to-work protocol, proceed with caution. It is very important to return to work as soon as you are medically stable and your doctor says it is safe for you to return. However, returning to work too soon can have disastrous consequences, the most serious of which is reinjury.

Remember: The case manager is not hired to be your friend or even your advocate. It may be easy for the case manager to gain your trust and confidence over time. Because your work with your case manager can go on for so long, it can *seem* like the case manager is your friend. Do not be fooled. She is not your friend any more than the adjustor who seems so sweet and caring is your friend. The case manager is hired by the insurance carrier. She is there to assist the communication between the team members involved in your care. Her job is to ensure that there are no delays in getting you back to work, or at the very least in obtaining documentation which shows that you have reached maximum medical improvement (MMI).

You are still your best advocate. It does not matter whether you have managed care insurance, workers' compensation or disability; the same applies to any case manager assigned to your claim. Unless you or your attorney hired the case manager for you, remember: She needs accurate, honest information; but never give her any information which you do not want everyone involved in your claim to have. You may have an excellent relationship with your case manager, but always remember who hired her and who pays her salary.

As a former MCM, I would advise you to request that the MCM meet with you and your doctor *after* the doctor has examined you. Unless the MCM was hired by you or your attorney, I would be cautious about inviting her into the room during your exam. I have heard doctors tell me one thing when I was a patient and afterwards tell the MCM something different. Those states that require your participation with medical case management do not usually require that the MCM be in the room during your exam, they just want to make sure that you cooperate with the MCM. You can cooperate with your MCM but not have her in the room during your personal physician's exam.

### Obtaining Authorizations

The MCM coordinates the authorization process between the doctors and providers and the insurance carrier for any various tests and procedures ordered. When a physician makes the authorization request for anything (e.g., surgery, medical equipment, therapy, etc.), there are specific guidelines which carriers have established to review the request before they will agree to pay for the procedure. The MCM can sometimes offer additional information—which may not have been documented in the physician's (provider's) request—thereby avoiding further delays.

Oftentimes, the doctor's office staff makes the call to request prior authorization. They may be working with very limited information at the time they place the call. An MCM can be extremely helpful by clarifying the need for the tests or procedures ordered. An MCM who has been working with you since the beginning of your claim has probably met with your physician and can provide the rationale for the request. This information would not normally be available to some administrative assistants making authorization calls. An effective case manager can expedite the authorization so that your care can keep moving forward. On the flip side of providing supportive information, the MCM can relay information to the carrier which will lead to a denial of the services requested. The MCM can provide her own opinions; if those opinions are contrary to your doctor's, the carrier may deny the requested test or procedure.

### Avoid Stiff Penalties

Your physician and his staff are well-acquainted with the need for obtaining prior authorization. Most healthcare providers have experienced reimbursement problems and have developed formal procedures to reduce their financial liabilities. They are aware that if they proceed without obtaining prior authorization they may not be paid. This does not pertain only to workers' compensation. If you are having any type of surgery or hospital admission, or require special assistive devices, I urge you to contact your insurance carrier directly. Most carriers—whether they are automobile liability, medical indemnity, managed care or disability carriers—will require some form of pre-certification or prior authorization. You may have a case manager working inside the company who can help you with this. You need to read the fine print in your policy and be in contact with your carrier to avoid possible stiff financial penalties.

## Ask Your Carrier For A Medical Case Manager

If you go ahead and have a procedure which has not been authorized and is not urgent or emergent, it could result in a denial of your claim. This could possibly mean that you will be stuck with the bill for the unauthorized procedure. If you have an MCM working on your claim, she can clarify what has been authorized. If the authorization has not been issued, she can ensure that it is processed. If you do not have a case manager, and the treatment plan is becoming quite extensive, and you have multiple providers, I would advise that you contact the carrier to see if it is possible that one can be assigned to your case. If an MCM is assigned at your request, just remember what was discussed before. You and your advocate need to continue to be part of the process.

## A Good Medical Case Manager

Having an MCM can be a tremendous benefit. Your MCM can make sure that you receive the care you need in a timely and efficient manner. She can also make sure that when you are released to return to work, the work that is available is safe for you.

Carol had been out of work for several months with a repetitive stress injury in her wrist. She had started to get better with the time away from her factory job. Prior to her MCM assignment, Carol had returned to work in what the employer felt was a suitable "light duty" position. Within a week of being back to work, Carol noticed that the pain, swelling and numbness had returned to her hands. It was obvious that although the work did not require heavy lifting, and was considered by the employer to be light duty, the work was repetitive and therefore unsuitable for Carol's condition. Carol returned to Dr. Stone, who immediately pulled her from work and made plans to do a surgical repair of her right arm. As soon as the carrier received Dr. Stone's request for the surgery, an MCM named Bobbie was assigned to the case. Bobbie met Carol at her first post-operative appointment with Dr. Stone. The carrier made it perfectly clear that they wanted Carol back at work as soon as possible.

Bobbie went to the employer and discussed Carol's restrictions. Dr. Stone agreed to release Carol back to light-duty work—as long as it did not involve any use of the right arm. Each job the employer offered was inappropriate. Bobbie decided the only way to make sure that Carol would be able to do the light duty work was to have her actually go and do the proposed job, using just her left hand. It immediately became evident that the light duty was not appropriate. Bobbie worked very closely with the employer and creatively developed a staggered return-to-work plan that met all the restrictions prescribed by Dr. Stone, and also fit the work that could be provided. Bobbie wrote up a Job Analysis (JA) and brought it to Dr. Stone. She requested that the work release be as specific as the JA which she had developed. This process was repeated each time Dr. Stone progressed Carol's work and relaxed her restrictions. Dr. Stone told Bobbie that he had never had an MCM be so specific, but he was pleased that Carol was able to transition back to work and remain at work without any further recurrent problems.

Bobbie was able to expedite each additional test and x-ray that Dr. Stone ordered. She was able to work with Carol's employer and coordinate a work schedule that would allow Carol to take breaks and leave to attend the required physical therapy sessions she needed to help her strengthen and regain the motion in her arm. Dr. Stone was so pleased with Bobbie's help on the case that he told several patients that they might want to request her for an MCM. Bobbie was open and honest with Carol, Dr. Stone, the employer and the carrier. She was able to make sure that Carol was not reinjured when she transitioned back to work. Bobbie was able to satisfy the carrier and employer and get Carol back to work sooner rather than later. Dr. Stone was very pleased that his staff did not have to spend months trying to get approval for follow-up MRI exams and therapy. Bobbie was the ideal in case management.

## The Medical Case Manager Will Not Lie For You

The nurse case manager is bound by a code of professional ethics. Do not try to place the case manager in a position to act in an unprofessional or untruthful manner. You can expect that if a problem is identified, the MCM will contact the appropriate members of the team to inform them and help prevent further complications. You need to remember that the MCM has been hired by the insurance carrier to coordinate your care and get you back to work as soon as possible. She will take whatever information you tell her and whatever she sees and pass it on to all members of your team. It is important, for example, that you understand if you are out of work for a back injury, and are receiving workers' compensation or disability benefits for that injury, and the case manager arrives to find you lifting heavy objects (including children or heavy pets) or climbing ladders, or performing activities outside of your prescribed restrictions, she is obligated to pass on this information to the members of your team. Such information will be given to the adjustor and it is very possible that it will be used to terminate your benefits or get a release for you to return to work.

If you have been instructed by your doctor to increase your activity and try to do as much as possible during the day, make sure that your doctor makes a note about this in your medical records. This documentation from your physician may help you continue to receive benefits. Unfortunately, a doctor may tell the patient that he wants her trying different chores around the house but does not mention this in his notes or to the case manager. Then if the MCM arrives or an investigator videotapes you mowing the lawn or doing other chores, it is often used to try to deny your benefits. This is yet another example of why you need to be involved in your care and know what is written in your records. You cannot appeal a denial of your benefits if you do not have all the information. Your doctor may tell you to try different activities to see how you feel afterwards; it helps him assess the progress you are making. If you do have a day when you feel especially good and are able to be more active, you should make a note about it in your personal binder—both so that you can discuss it with your doctor and also to help you should it become an issue later. There is no good justification for not keeping track of, and writing down, absolutely everything. The stakes are very high; your future compensation or disability benefits may depend on what you do.

## Exploring Your Options

If you have questions about the MCM's role in your situation, you should first speak with the insurance carrier. If you are in the workers' compensation system, you should clarify the issues with the state regulating agency. If you do not want to work with an MCM, you will need to find out from your state or federal agency if refusing this service is an option. Many states have adopted laws which make participation with medical case management mandatory. In those states, failure to cooperate with the medical case manager can result in a termination or denial of your benefits. Carriers in states which do not have mandatory participation regulations may have instructed their adjustors to assign a case manager for specific injuries or diagnoses, or for claimants who have been out of work for a certain period of time.

If you are working with an MCM who you feel places the interests of the insurance carrier before yours, contact an attorney to determine how you should handle the situation. The MCM does not need to be your friend or advocate, but neither should the MCM be an adversary. It is very important if you are working with an MCM that you understand what your rights are in regards to that relationship. If you feel there is a conflict of interest, or you do not want to work with the case manager for some other reason, you must address this issue. Under favorable circumstances, the medial case manager can be an excellent resource.

## Things To Remember

- Get to know the Medical Case Manager if you have one.
- Understand for whom the Medical Case Manager works.
- Make sure you understand what is said to you by your providers and case manager.
- Make sure that you are copied on all of the case manager's reports.
- Be aware of what information the MCM is providing to the other members of your team.
- Remember: The MCM is not hired to be your friend.

- Enlist the case manager to expedite your care and authorizations.
- Do not expect the MCM to lie or cover for you.
- Know your options regarding working with, or firing, the MCM.

## Questions You Need To Ask

- Who is my Medical Case Manager? Is the case manager a vocational or medical professional?
- Who hired my MCM? What role is she expected to play?
- Are there laws that regulate if I must work with an MCM? What penalties will I face if I refuse?
- Has the MCM provided me with copies of all papers which I signed, and all reports and correspondences she has written and submitted regarding my care?
- If I have a complicated illness or injury, have I contacted the carrier to inquire about having a case manager available to assist with coordination of my care?

# 12

## *Vocational Rehabilitation*

**W**orking for years in a profession or job you love can be immensely satisfying. It puts food on your table and gives you the pride of being productive. But what happens when you lose your job because you are too sick or disabled to return to that position? What happens if you lack the education or alternate ways to earn an income? What happens if all you know is hard labor and now you can only work in a sedentary job, but have no skills to make the change? What happens when your illness impairs your ability to work full-time, and you are able to work part-time but there is no such job available? All of these questions can be answered by a referral for a Vocational Rehabilitation assessment.

### What Is Vocational Rehabilitation?

Vocational Rehabilitation (Voc Rehab) is the process by which a specialist works with an injured or ill individual to assist him in locating, obtaining and sustaining gainful employment. The term vocational can be used to mean something that is related to a person's job, career or profession. The Voc Rehab case manager can perform an assessment to see what the individual is physically and vocationally capable of doing. Voc Rehab is a process that is regulated by professional licensure boards, workers' compensation or the insurance industry in each individual state. Each state has differing rules and regulations which apply to the practice and application of Voc Rehab to their claimants receiving compensation or disability benefits. If you have been out of work for more than four weeks, or if you have experienced a disability or illness which has displaced you from your previous job, contact your state agency to see if there are any Voc Rehab services you might be entitled to receive.

### The Entitlement Assessment

Some states mandate that claimants who have been out of work for a specific amount of time must have a vocational entitlement assessment. A Voc Rehab counselor or case manager will meet with you to review your current medical condition, your past work history, your current work status (including your current status with your employer), and your future employment options. The entitlement process can be lengthy. Oftentimes if the claimant is still too injured or ill to make a determination, the Voc Rehab counselor may delay making the decision about the entitlement for, or appropriateness of services. The entitlement assessment will help the members of your team determine if there are other options for your return to work. The entitlement assessment can help you understand what your future employment might look like.

### Federal Agencies And Voc Rehab

Voc Rehab services were addressed by the federal government when it passed the Rehabilitation Act of 1973. This was the first legislation passed which addressed the vocational needs of and discrimination against disabled individuals. The act was later amended in 1992 (see Appendix C). The federal government also established the Office of Special Education and Rehabilitation Services (OSERS), which is committed to making sure that people with disabilities reach their maximum functional potential. Voc Rehab can be very expensive. These services are not consistently offered from state to state for workers' compensation claimants. If you live in a state which does not require any formal Voc Rehab services for individuals in the workers' compensation system, contact other state-sponsored and private, local career and vocational vendors. If you are not sure where to find them, check in the yellow pages under "Career and Vocational Counselors," or contact your local Department of Labor. The Department of Labor or "Employment Office" can be very helpful. These agencies are staffed with individuals trained and certified to address various vocational issues.

## Not Everyone Is Entitled

Once you call or are contacted by a Voc Rehab counselor to assist you with your vocational needs, proceed with caution. Do not assume that if you are to have a mandatory vocational entitlement assessment that you will automatically be found entitled. Do not assume that the Voc Rehab counselor contracted by the workers' compensation carrier will be completely unbiased and advocate for services for you. There are many factors which will play a role in determining your eligibility. Do not assume that just because you are unable to return to your former employer due to your condition that you will automatically be found entitled.

## The Vocational Assessment

When you have a Vocational Assessment, the counselor will do an extensive review of your medical history, including reviewing your medical records. He may also address any complicating psychological issues which may impact your Voc Rehab. It is important that the vocational case manager have an accurate picture of your desire to return to work. He or she will contact your employer to review your current work and employment status with them. The counselor will take a detailed work history which will include where you worked, what jobs you had and how much money you made. He will want to know about your educational history. These work and educational histories will be used to determine if you have any transferable skills. Transferable skills are those that can be used in another job (in the event that you will not be returning to your previous position). The counselor will contact your treating physician to discuss the various options and prognosis for your return to work.

## You May Need A New Employer

The ideal expectation is for you to return to your previous employer, but this may not be an option for several reasons. If you have been terminated (fired or let go) by your employer and there is no longer a position available to you, do not assume that this will automatically entitle you to Voc Rehab services. Not all states require that your employer hold your position for you. Some have specific requirements that address your right to another job within the company. If your injury is work-related, be sure to check with your state workers' compensation division to understand your rights. Each state is different. There are a multitude of factors that will impact the entitlement process. If you are a person with transferable skills, and therefore will not require a lot of retraining or schooling, it is possible that you may not be found entitled. If you are not entitled to Voc Rehab services and have reached MMI you will be expected to find a new job on your own, without the help of a Voc Rehab specialist. The states all have various rules and regulations which address this. If you have questions, contact your state agency or your lawyer for clarification of the laws.

If you are out of work on a non-work-related illness or injury, and are using disability benefits or benefits related to the Family and Medical Leave Act of 1993 (FMLA), you will need to go through the same process. You will need to clarify what the company's policies are. You will also need to contact the carrier or search the Department of Labor's website to clarify what your rights and responsibilities are under FMLA (see Appendix C). There are some employers who will offer their employees use of the FMLA benefits if they are trying to help their employee maintain their position within the company. This can be especially true if the employer knows that the employee will be returning to work within the twelve-week FMLA period. If you intend to apply for FMLA leave, make sure you check with your human resources representative to clarify what you will need to do to ensure that you will have a job awaiting your return. This can be very important, especially if you want to use FMLA time as an intermittent benefit.

If you are out of work for a non-work-related illness or injury and you do not have a contract protecting your position, there is no guarantee that your employer will hold your position—or take you back in another position—once you are released to return to work. Most companies will offer their employees some sick leave. This can vary from company to company. It can also vary within the company, depending upon your title and/or job responsibilities. Companies can claim they provide a couple of weeks of sick time; however, these same companies might write you up or reprimand you for using the sick time which is supposed to be a benefit. Do not assume that just because your employer offers ten sick days a year that they will be okay with you using all ten days. Make sure you understand your company policies or your contract before you rush to use all of your sick time. Some companies still require notes from your doctor if you are going to use a certain number of days of your sick time.

### For Whom Does The Voc Rehab Case Manager Work?

Depending on where you live and which state has jurisdiction over your claim, if you are found to be entitled to Voc Rehab services, the state may have strict regulations regarding who can be a Voc Rehab case manager. As with MCMs, Voc Rehab counselors can work for the state agency, a private corporation, be self-employed, or be part of the service provided by your workers' compensation carrier. Some Voc Rehab counselors work with attorneys to help them determine what financial losses their clients suffered with the loss of their jobs or ability to return to any job. Some large employers hire Voc Rehab counselors to work with their employees as they develop a return-to-work plan. As with MCMs, Voc Rehab counselors can be strong advocates who ensure that you have the best services available.

On the other hand, they might work for companies that promise the carriers a specific percentage of their claimants will not be found "Not Entitled." This may mean they are completing assessments that are inaccurate or incomplete, and are doomed before they are started. These counselors are hired by carriers to make sure that some claimants are not found to be entitled to Voc Rehab services. Voc Rehab is an expensive process and can result in increased workers' compensation premiums. If you have concerns about the Voc Rehab counselor with whom you are working, discuss this with your attorney.

### The Comprehensive Voc Rehab Plan

If you are entitled to Voc Rehab services, you will begin working closely with your counselor to develop a comprehensive plan. You will work with the counselor to review local employment options, set goals and identify your strengths and weaknesses. You may take aptitude and placement tests to help identify for what employment you might be best suited, especially if you are unable to return to the type of work that you did previously. You may take some simple tests to help you and the counselor see what your educational abilities are. The Voc Rehab counselor will work with you, local employers and possibly your previous employer to identify appropriate job opportunities you might pursue. You will revamp or complete a resume and you may be given coaching techniques to assist you in the interview process when you apply for a job.

### The Functional Capacity Evaluation (FCE)

The Voc Rehab counselor may contact your physician to see if you should have a Functional Capacity Evaluation (FCE) to determine your current physical capabilities. The FCE will also identify if additional work hardening and/or physical and occupational therapy might help you find a job that is more physically challenging. An FCE can be very useful to your physician as he signs your final work release. The FCE can identify ongoing weaknesses and problem areas which indicate a need for permanent restrictions. If you are scheduled for an FCE, you can be sure that it will be a fairly grueling test of your physical ability.

The best FCE is an objective test. Many facilities offer Functional Capacity testing, but they are unsophisticated and the administrator of the test relies on your subjective complaints and her personal observations. The most objective FCE is based on a computerized testing model which can assess your actual ability, as well as the effort you put into the test. It does not rely on the personal opinion of the test administrator. The people administering the FCE can objectively assess certain signs that indicate your body is putting forth a lot of effort. Clients who go through the testing with only minimal effort can have a negative FCE which is false and inaccurate. This in turn can have a negative impact on your Voc Rehab options, as well as a negative impact on your permanent partial impairment. If you feel that putting forth minimal effort during the test will somehow benefit you financially at a future time, you are mistaken. Effort and exertion can be assessed. If the test administrator sees that you have not put forth the effort and the test results confirm that you did not work to your ability—regardless of your limitations—this information will be included in the report and may negatively impact your future claim.

## The FCE Can Help

If you have put forth all of the effort that you can, and it is evident that with more physical rehabilitation your situation can improve, your physician may change your current treatment plan. It is important to remember that your doctor will ultimately receive the copy of the FCE report. The physician will be able to interpret the results and recommendations from the testing summary and make further determinations about your needs. It may also help him determine if you have reached MMI (maximum medical improvement—the point in your illness or injury there is no additional improvement expected from the additional treatment). The FCE can be a valuable tool as you begin to make your job search list with your Voc Rehab counselor. It will help you identify jobs that you are physically capable of performing. If the test identifies that you are only able to do sedentary or light work as established by the United States Department of Labor, it will do you no good to be looking for jobs that require heavy work endurance and physical ability.

## The Difficult Adjustment

Once you have recovered from your injury or illness, you may not be able to return to your former occupation. It will be necessary for you to work closely with your Voc Rehab counselor to identify positions that are suited to your physical, mental and vocational abilities. It can be an especially difficult challenge to find a new job that satisfies you the way your previous job did. It can be demoralizing and frustrating to try to be happy in a new job when a large part of who you are was related to what you were able to do before the accident or illness. This can be especially true for the person who worked for many years as a loyal employee of a company, and now finds that she is unable to return to the company and her former job.

Margaret had been participating in a multidisciplinary rehabilitation program with the hope that she would be able to return to her preinjury position as a Floor Manager for a large warehouse supply store. Her job had heavy physical demands, requiring frequent heavy lifting of weights in excess of fifty to sixty pounds. It required her to be on her feet for several hours at a time, with prolonged periods of standing and walking. She had tried to work part-time and attend physical therapy sessions a couple of times each week; however, her symptoms worsened and she was eventually taken out of work completely so that she could participate in the rehabilitation program. Unfortunately, her symptoms worsened and she was unable to return to the department which she loved—dashing her hopes of advancing to the position of Store Manager. It seemed to Margaret that her employer took great enjoyment in the termination of her position. She was told that she could return if she could meet the physical requirements, but given her injury and deteriorating condition, she was not able to return.

Margaret felt isolated and abandoned by everyone at work. Compounding her physical isolation was a feeling of social isolation, and eventually, sadness and frustration. In spite of excellent performance reviews at work, she felt that her employer was simply looking for a way to terminate their working relationship and reduce their liability. They knew that if Margaret returned to work there was a good possibility of another injury or extended time away from work, which would cost them a large amount of money again. Her company was looking out for themselves, not Margaret.

Feelings of frustration and anger can become even more prominent if the injured worker feels like her employer was anxious to get rid of her. If you find that you are suffering from anxiety and depression related to your new changes, it is important to let your doctor or Voc Rehab counselor know about it. Perhaps you may need some additional counseling to help you with your adjustment. There is a certain level of stress when a person *voluntarily* changes jobs, but the level of stress can be magnified if the person feels the change was forced upon her.

### You Are Integral To The Voc Rehab Plan

You need to take control of the Vocational Rehabilitation plan that you develop with your counselor. You will not have a successful plan if you do not feel involved and in control. No one can tell you what job you must do. Your counselor can suggest various options, but if it is something that does not interest you, do not waste your time looking into it. If you are looking at jobs that involve retraining—and possibly relocating—you should also check to see if funds are available to help you train and/or move. If you have a workers' compensation claim open, you will want to see if you qualify for lost wages, travel expenses, tuition and books, and possibly even start-up fees if you are considering self-employment. Some states do not approve self-employment plans as a Voc Rehab alternative. If you want to be retrained, the retraining should be reasonable; for example, do not expect that you will be sent to an expensive college if you have not yet received your GED or high school diploma. You may be entitled to retraining, but you might not be sent to college if you have never had any training outside of high school. An injury or illness is not a guarantee of an all-expenses-paid, four-year degree.

### What About Special Accommodations?

Once you find a job that might possibly be right for you, your counselor can complete a job analysis and possibly an ergonomic assessment to make sure that the physical demands and job environment meet your abilities. The job analysis can be reviewed by your doctor to make sure that the job is appropriate and safe for you, physically. Your potential new employer may be willing to make certain modifications to your new work station which would make it more suitable to your physical needs.

The Americans with Disabilities Act (ADA) addresses the issues of "reasonable accommodations." The ADA requires that employers who have fifteen or more employees provide reasonable accommodations to help their employees with disabilities do their jobs. If an employee hopes that her employer will accommodate her physical or mental limitations, she must be honest with her employer about those limitations. This does *not* mean that an employer is obligated to hire someone who is unqualified to do the job and then provide another person to help her complete the essential tasks of the job. The ADA defines something that is reasonable as that which is "achievable" and will allow a qualified person to perform the job in spite of her limitations. For further clarification of the ADA regulations go to their website (see Appendix C). You will need to clarify with your counselor—and possibly your lawyer—what changes would constitute a reasonable accommodation. Your counselor may also check with your previous employer to see if they are willing to make certain accommodations, allowing you to return to your old position.

### Start Your Own Search

If you are unable to return to your previous position and you 1) have reached maximum medical improvement, 2) have been given a release to return to work and 3) are not entitled to Voc Rehab services under your workers' compensation claim, you will have to begin your own job search. You can still be receiving workers' compensation benefits and be terminated from a work position in some states. It is not always a smart thing for an employer to terminate an employee who is out of work with an ongoing workers' compensation claim; bringing an employee back for a certain time (established by the state) or offering them light duty or transitional work can help reduce the employer's workers' compensation premiums when it comes time for renewal of their policy. Some carriers have specific clauses in their contracts which require employers to provide transitional or light-duty work for their employees. Some states require an employer to make every effort to bring an employee back to work; then after a certain time period, if there are personnel issues not related to the workers' compensation claim, the employer may terminate the employee. Just because a person is receiving workers' compensation benefits does not mean his employment is guaranteed. There are some employers who will terminate an employee after just a few days out of work. They might send their employee a certified letter informing him of the termination, or they might just give him a call and let him know that he is no longer working for the company.

It would be nice to believe that an employer cannot fire you while you are out of work, whether for a work-related or non-work-related illness or injury. But unless you have a contract for employment, most employers will do what they want—even if they are threatened with a suit for wrongfully terminating/discharging an employee. If you are receiving workers' compensation benefits and you are terminated, you should check with your local Department of Labor to see how and when you can qualify for unemployment benefits. You should also ask about their Voc Rehab services. If you are out of work for a non-work-related claim and are terminated, you will still need to call the Department of Labor. You might need the services of the Department of Labor to help you find another job if you are planning to return to work after your recovery. A good rule of thumb is to contact the Department of Labor as soon as you find out that you have been fired or terminated. If you hear rumors that you might be terminated, call the Department of Labor proactively to determine what your options are.

If you belonged to a union prior to your injury, you will want to contact your union representative for assistance in helping you locate a new job. The other alternative is to investigate agencies in your area that offer temporary employment opportunities. They sometimes have temporary assignments which transition to permanent positions and offer benefits. Various state laws will say how a work slow-down or lay-off will affect your workers' compensation or disability benefits if you are released to return to work during the lay-off period.

## Restrictions And Limitations

Once you find a job, you will want to make sure that the physical demands of that job comply with any physical restrictions prescribed by your doctor. Some workers will take a position knowing full well that they might be reinjured and have to be out of work again. Some do this to try to keep their place with the company, while others do it hoping that they will receive compensation or disability benefits to stay home again. The laws can be very specific about what happens in this situation. The laws are also specific about defining the reinjury as a new injury or an aggravation. If it appears as though the problem that you develop is an extension of your previous claim, there is no guarantee that you will be entitled to benefits again. The laws in each state are specific about when and for what reasons a claim can be reopened. Once you find a job—whether on your own or with the help of a vocational counselor—your vocational case management might not be complete. Your vocational case manager may stay in touch with you for a period of time to make sure that you do not have any complications once you return to work. It is important to keep those lines of communication open.

## Talking To Prospective New Employers

You should talk to your vocational counselor and your lawyer about what to tell a potential new employer concerning your recent injury or illness. The laws are specific and generally prevent potential employers from asking about your health during the application or interview process. There are some people who readily share this information during their interviews. This can sometimes work to your advantage; the prospective employer may feel that you are open and honest and someone they would like to hire. In other cases, being too honest about a disability can backfire. Telling a prospective employer that you really cannot do the job because of a recent or ongoing treatment for an injury can eliminate any chance you might have of getting the position. If you are trying to avoid returning to work and deliberately offer information about your disability in hopes of sabotaging an employment offer, you will soon find that your vocational options decrease—possibly along with your compensation or disability benefits. Whether you should discuss a disability with a potential employer is a complex issue and should be handled on a case-by-case basis, as there really does not seem to be a standard way to proceed.

### The Voc Rehab Report

As with everything else related to your injury or illness, you should obtain copies of all Voc Rehab case manager reports and correspondence. Most vocational case managers will copy you on letters that they send out, but some will not. It is up to you to make sure that you get the copies and add them to your binder. Once you receive the Voc Rehab reports, be sure to read them. If you have questions about anything in the reports, bring it to the attention of the case manager or your attorney. This can be especially important if the case manager determines that you are not entitled to Voc Rehab services. If your state has laws which provide for vocational rehab services and you feel that you were unjustly denied these services, file an appeal with the state regulating agency. Remember that the vocational case manager is usually hired by the carrier and may try save money for the carrier by finding you not entitled to services. Voc Rehab case managers are not your friends; they are hired to do a job.

### Changing Case Managers

As with your Medical Case Manager, if you are dissatisfied with your Voc Rehab case manager you should check with your carrier to see if being referred to another vocational case manager is an option. If this is a work-related claim, the state workers' compensation division can tell you what your rights are. Not all states require that a Voc Rehab assessment and plan be in place. Those that do, have specific regulations to address how to proceed if you want a new case manager. In some states, case managers work independently and are not part of a larger case management company. If your vocational case manager works for a larger company and you are simply swapping one of their employees for another, you might not be much happier than you were before. Both of these employees are working under the same company policies and may operate similarly. On the other hand, if your case manager is an independent subcontractor, check with your carrier to see if they have another person to whom they can refer you. If you have a lawyer, make sure to check with him. Lawyers usually have a referral list of vocational and/or medical case managers with whom they want their clients working. In general, lawyers should have a good idea of which vocational case managers will work for you and which ones will work to benefit your carrier.

### Being Your Own Vocational Case Manager

You will know when you are ready to return to work if you have a physician who keeps you informed of your progress. It is up to you to ask how you are coming along and what you can expect. Be sure to ask when you can begin planning to go back to work. If your doctor tells you that you will be ready in a certain amount of time, you can count on that as being the maximum time it might take. If you are motivated, you might be able to speed up the process and see if you can go back to work sooner with some restrictions. If you are ready to return to work and you do not have a workers' compensation claim, or you work in a state that does not provide Voc Rehab services, you might have to be your own vocational case manager. If you are going back to your preinjury/illness employer, you will want to maintain an open line of communication the entire time you are out of work. Your employer will need to know if you are released for light duty, or if you are coming back to full duty without restrictions.

If you are not going back to your former employer and need to start a job search, seek out as many resources as possible. Be sure to get the word out and network, letting people know that you are in the market for a new job. Check with your local Department of Labor to see if there are any incentive programs, such as a job training program, for which you might qualify. Check to see if your local Chamber of Commerce has any leads, offers, retraining and/or new employment bonuses for local employers to hire new staff. Check your phone directory for vocational counselors to see if there might be one who can work with you using money put aside by the state to retrain displaced workers. Check out any local agencies for individuals with disabilities. These agencies can make all the difference in ensuring your successful return to work and adaptation to any permanent disabilities you might have.

## Things To Remember

- Vocational Rehabilitation is not just for injured workers.
- Call the carrier to see if they will cover an entitlement assessment.
- There are federal laws and services which regulate and provide for Voc Rehab.
- The vocational assessment addresses all issues surrounding your disability.
- Clarify who your vocational case manager is and for whom he works
- You may need a Functional Capacity Evaluation before a plan can be made.
- An objective FCE is vital for your safety and health.
- The vocational case manager can be instrumental in clarifying your restrictions and coordinating the accommodations you may need.
- Not everyone with a disability or injury is entitled to Voc Rehab.
- If you are found to be not entitled, you may have to find your own new job.
- Make sure your new job fits your restrictions and limitations.

## Questions You Need To Ask

- Who is my vocational case manager?
- For whom does my vocational case manager work? Who pays for his services and the assessment? Is there a potential conflict of interest?
- Is a vocational case manager assessment and intervention mandatory to my claim?
- What is a Vocational Entitlement Assessment? Do I need one? How will it affect my situation?
- What happens if I am not entitled?
- Do I have a copy of my Voc Rehab plan and copies of updated reports from my vocational case manager?
- Are there other resources available that can help me with the Voc Rehab process?
- Can I change vocational case managers if I am dissatisfied with my current case manager?
- If I have special needs and restrictions, who will assist me with the accommodations that I need if and when I return to work?
- Should I tell potential employers about my disabilities?

**13**

## *Return To Work*

**R**eturning to work can be an exciting part of your rehabilitation. For others, it is the one part of their injury and rehabilitation that they would like to avoid—it is easier for them to stay home and collect a paycheck (compensation check, disability check, or unemployment check). There are some patients who are permanently and totally disabled who will never return to work. This chapter is for those patients who have been released to return to work.

### Are You Able To Return to Work?

Whether you are currently working with a Voc Rehab counselor or not, the issue of when you are able to return to work is sure to arise. Unless you have been declared permanently totally disabled, you will eventually be released to return to work. Whether or not you return to work full duty or with restrictions will be up to your doctor. If you have been declared totally disabled due to a severe injury or illness you will not return to work and will most likely apply for Social Security Disability Income (SSDI). Applying for SSDI benefits is a complex process and can take several months or longer. If you have questions regarding permanent disability and SSDI benefits, contact your local Social Security Office and/or your attorney.

### Transitional Work Assignments

For purposes of this book, it is assumed that you will be released to return to work once you are medically stable and have regained enough strength to meet the various physical requirements of your job or an alternate job. If you have not regained your preinjury or pre-illness strength and endurance, you may be released to return to work in a transitional position. A transitional position is one that is considered temporary and allows you to transition or return to work at a slower pace. If you are a claimant in a workers' compensation or disability system, it is likely that the contract the insurance carrier has with your employer mandates some form of return-to-work policy. Many contracts will specify that if there is a release for work with restrictions, the employer must make an effort to accommodate these restrictions for the injured worker. Most employers will make every effort to find some type of transitional or light-duty work for their employee. Some employers will not. You will need to check with your state agency to clarify the laws regarding whether your employer must offer transitional work duties.

### Make Sure The Release Is Specific

If you are released to return to some form of work, it is important to be very sure that your physician makes the release as explicit as possible. When a physician writes, "May return to light-duty work" or "Light-Duty Work," it could open the door to many problems. It is very important to have the release specifically identify the various tasks of which you are and are not capable. If you have a release, you will want the doctor to clearly state how long you can work, what activities you can and cannot do, and if you have any activity restrictions or other physical limitations that will impede your work. Ask your doctor to make the release as detailed as possible.

## Light Duty Is Not Always Light Duty

When an employee comes to the employer with a work release that simply offers the statement "Light-Duty Work," it can cause a lot of problems for the employee. Consider, for example, a person who has been away from his job on the assembly line in a factory with a repetitive stress injury in his arm. There are many employers who insist that the work on the assembly line is "light" duty. They assume that because the parts that the employee handles over and over are light*weight* that this means the position is automatically light duty. They believe that it will be acceptable for the employee because it does not require "heavy" work. Or, they may move the employee to another part of the plant where they have him move small objects through a machine or place them in small bags repetitively throughout the shift. All of this work requires repetitive motions—the very sort of activity that caused the injury. It can take a tremendous amount of work to educate employers on repetitive activities, and these tasks—which are "light" in terms of weight—are actually "heavy" in duty. Most likely, at this stage of your recovery you are working with an MCM or a Voc Rehab counselor. If so, she should make sure that your release is appropriate and the assigned duties meet your release restrictions and will not cause additional problems or another injury.

## A Job Analysis Is Crucial

For those of you who are managing your own care, when you are ready to return to work, it is a good idea to call your Human Resources representative and request a copy of both your job description and a copy of your job analysis. A job analysis is a summary of all of the tasks that make up your job, and breaks down the physical tasks into the total number of hours spent during the day. It addresses the total number of hours worked, the number of breaks assigned and the essential and non-essential tasks to be performed. If your employer states that a job analysis does not exist, make a list of all the tasks which you perform during your shift. Review this list with your doctor to make sure that no aspect of your job will conflict with any prescribed restrictions. The job analysis can be used as a guide to set your recovery goals. This is especially true if you are planning to return to your previous job. It also can be a good summary of what led to your current injury or problem.

## A Staggered Return To Work Plan Can Be Successful

You might also benefit from a staggered (gradual) return to work schedule. Your medical case manager should try to coordinate with your employer to plan a return to work with incrementally increasing hours over the first few weeks—especially if you have permanent physical limitations. Clients have the most success with their return to work when they return perhaps for two to four hours a day for the first few days or weeks and then gradually add hours and duties. Most people who are out of work for prolonged periods of time become physically deconditioned. Even those who have attended physical therapy on a regular basis may struggle their first couple of weeks back to work. There are individuals who are strong and physically able to return full-time, full-duty; but for those who are not, a staggered work release with incremental time and task increases is a better option. Staggering a return to work is a safe, effective way to reintegrate the worker back at the job without aggravating his original injury or putting him at risk for another injury.

## Return To Work Problems

There are some people who are very reluctant to return to work with a light-duty work release. Most often, the injured worker has seen coworkers return to what was termed a light-duty position, only to have the work nearly identical to the work that contributed to his original injury. He may have seen how some people are ridiculed by their coworkers, or embarrassed by their supervisors when they return to a transitional-duty position. Regardless of the reason for your reluctance, if you are part of a workers' compensation or disability program and you have been given a release to return to work, and your employer can accommodate your return, you will have to return to work. If you refuse light-duty work or work which your doctor says you are capable of doing, you risk immediate termination of your benefits. If you feel that the work which is offered does not meet the restrictions prescribed by your physician, you will have to contact your physician, an attorney, or the regulating agency or carrier to intervene. Do not just fail to show up without talking to someone about your concerns.

### Some Benefits May Continue

People who are placed in a transitional position are often very concerned that their workers' compensation or disability benefits will terminate. In some states, if your return to work is on a part-time basis, a percentage of your benefits may supplement your reduced wages. You will need to clarify what your benefits will be with your state agency and carrier. If you are working part-time and are able to obtain partial workers' compensation benefits to offset your part-time hours, you should be in contact with the insurance carrier to determine how they will handle this. You will want to know if your checks will continue with the same regularity with which they had been coming or if there will be a delay. It is important to clarify this—especially if you are counting on that check to pay bills. Some carriers request that the employer submit copies of payroll records, while others request that you submit a copy of your pay stub. If you send a copy of your pay stub, make sure to keep a copy for yourself. You must continue to keep meticulous records in case there is a dispute about the benefits owed to you. Keep track of the time that you work and what you are paid to offset your reduced wages. Be sure to call if you notice a discrepancy. Do not wait for several checks to see if the money "catches up." Keep an accurate record of those to whom you talked and when you talked to them. Make a note of what was discussed. If you feel that you are not being paid what is due to you, call your lawyer. If you are out of work for a long period of time, you might also be entitled to a cost-of-living increase in your compensation checks.

### What About Fringe Benefits?

If you are not working—whether it is a workers' compensation absence or one related to a medical, long-term disability—you should check with your employer to see what happens to your benefits while you are out of work. Do not assume that because you are out of work for a work-related illness or injury your employer will continue to pay for your benefits. Do not assume that you will continue to accrue vacation or sick time. Do not assume that your retirement contributions will continue. This also applies to work absences that are not related to your employment, but might keep you out for more than just a few days or weeks. Most companies are trying to streamline their budgets and one way they can do this is by suspending their contributions for your benefits (such as your health, disability or life insurance, and retirement accounts). Many do not allow employees who are out of work for specified extended periods of time continue to accrue vacation or sick time. Most companies clearly outline these rules in their policy manuals. If you work for a smaller company that does not have a policy manual, once you clarify with your employer what happens to your benefits, you should send a letter to the person with whom you talked to confirm your understanding. This can be especially important if you are hoping to take an extended vacation, based on accrued time, after you return to work. Most states do not regulate what employers must do with benefits when their employees are out of work.

### Working "Under the Table" Is Fraudulent

Trying to supplement reduced weekly paychecks by taking on a part-time job or by working "under the table" when you are unable to do your own job is fraudulent, and can lead to large fines and criminal prosecution. Most state insurance regulating agencies have fraud units designed specifically to deal with people who are receiving insurance (compensation or disability) benefits when they are capable of working. Insurance fraud carries stiff penalties. Not only can you be fined, but you could be required to pay back any or all of the compensation that you received.

## Know Your Restrictions And Adhere To Them

Once you are on your way back to work, it is very important that you understand exactly what your restrictions are. It will be your responsibility to make sure that you adhere to the restrictions prescribed by your doctor. If your employer or supervisor has you doing work outside of your restrictions, you must address this immediately. If you choose to do work outside of your restrictions, you must stop immediately. In either instance, working outside of your restrictions—either by direction of your supervisor or by your own choice—means that if you file a claim for an additional injury as a result of this activity, it is possible that the carrier will deny the claim. If your employer provides a light-duty assignment which strictly follows your physician's orders, and you choose to work outside of that position—either by helping out a coworker, or doing a task which is not assigned to you—your position with the company could be challenged, as you are doing work which you technically are not hired to do at that time. Some employers will take strong disciplinary action (including termination) with employees who are supposed to be following light-duty restrictions, but who take it upon themselves to do tasks from their preinjury position. If you feel that you are able to do more than what you are currently released to do, speak with your physician and have the restrictions removed or changed.

## Transitional Duty Is Not Permanent

As you progress with your transitional duty assignment, you should understand that each state has its own guidelines about transitional duty. Most states do not require your employer to give you a light-duty position or create a position for you. If you are given a transitional duty position, it is with the understanding that the position is temporary. Transitional duty work is not provided for an indefinite period of time. If you feel that the current duties you are performing are the most you will be able or want to do, you need to speak with your employer. Most employers may make accommodations for you for a few months, but it is not reasonable for you to expect they will offer this work permanently. Most transitional-duty jobs are new positions created to meet the current need of the injured worker. It is likely that your employer is expecting you to return to your original position at some time in the near future. If you do not want to return to your preinjury position, you need to look for another job.

## What About Another Position?

Some states have regulations which say that if you cannot return to your original preinjury position, the company must offer you the first available position which meets your capabilities. There is usually a time restriction on this; for example, a state might say you have the right to be offered a position for which you are qualified within two years from the onset of disability. This is a very confusing statement as it can be interpreted in two ways. It can be taken to mean that the two years begin at the time of your injury. It could also mean that the two years commences the first day that you are unable to perform your duties. Some adjustors will try to interpret these laws in whichever way will save the company more money.

If you need clarification, you are advised to discuss this with your attorney. As with other portions of the disability and workers' compensation systems, these guidelines vary from state to state. Insurance carriers are bound by the laws of the state in which they manage their claims. Many carriers have their main offices in one state but manage claims for several states. If you feel you have an issue with a carrier regarding your rights to return to work and the amount of compensation you are to receive, call your state agency or your lawyer.

## Make Sure The Release Is Individualized

When you are released to return to work, obtain a copy of the work release signed by your physician. If there is an associated job analysis which clearly identifies the various aspects of your job, have a copy of this signed by your doctor as well. Read over your job analysis and be sure that both you and your physician understand all of the physical demands and exposures associated with your job. If you have questions or concerns, make sure that your physician addresses these before you return to work. In addition to the signed work release and signed job analysis, be sure to remember to get a copy of your doctor's note. Check to make sure that he did not write one thing in his note but another on your work release.

## What If It Is Too Difficult To Work?

It is not unusual to hear that some people are not able to return to work as originally planned. If you are released to return to work and you find that once you have returned, you experience a recurrence of your symptoms or a worsening of your condition, you should immediately notify your supervisor and Human Resources representative. Next, you should contact your doctor and make a follow-up appointment as soon as one is available. Do not be surprised if your doctor cannot see you right away in the office. Some will refer their patients to the emergency room to make sure that there is not a new or acute problem that needs immediate attention.

If you are taken out of work again, make sure to continue to document your condition and contacts just as you did before you returned to work. If you maintain open lines of communication with your employer, it is possible they might be able to provide you with an alternate work assignment. On the other hand, if your employer is not interested in your welfare and insists on no changes to your routine, be sure to reconnect with your physician as soon as possible and let him intervene for you. If you are working with a case manager, also give her a call and let her assess the situation. Make sure to also notify your carrier. The last thing a carrier wants is to pay for a reinjury or another extended time out of work. If you have an attorney, notify him of the situation as well.

If you have a Medical Case Manager, you can request that she intervene with your employer to perform an ergonomic work-site assessment. This ergonomic assessment evaluates your work station, whether it is a desk, spot on a factory assembly line or even a check-out cashier's station. The ergonomic assessment will be used to make sure that your work area provides you the optimal positioning and posture while you perform your job duties. The person performing the ergonomic assessment is trained to evaluate each individual work station for the individual worker. Simple changes to the placement of items used to perform your job can help alleviate discomfort and may ultimately help you stay at work and be more comfortable doing your job.

If you are very uncomfortable and feel that you cannot continue working, make sure to have your physician provide an excuse that takes you out of work again until you can see him for a re-evaluation. Do not just walk off the job. *You* might know that you are leaving because you are too ill or in too much pain to be there, but leaving without following through with the appropriate procedures of notification could make it appear that you have quit your job.

### *Things To Remember*

- Make sure the return-to-work release is explicit.
- Light-duty work is not always "light duty."
- Obtain the job analysis to identify the actual physical tasks of the job.
- Investigate a staggered return-to-work option.
- An incremental increase in your tasks can be safer.
- Refusing a position can jeopardize your benefits.
- You may receive partial benefits.
- Know your restrictions and follow them.
- Working "under the table" is fraudulent and illegal.
- Transitional duty is not permanent.
- You may have to find another job and a new employer.

- Have I been released to return to work?
- Do I have a specific list of my return-to-work restrictions?
- Are my restrictions compatible with the job analysis for my work?
- How long will I have these restrictions? How long will I have to do a light-duty or transitional work assignment?
- If I return to work part time, will my benefits offset the reduced earnings?
- What happens if I refuse light duty or transitional work if it meets my restrictions?
- What should I do if I am "forced" by my employer to perform work duties that exceed my restrictions?
- What happens if I am reinjured or my symptoms worsen when I return to work?
- While I am out of work, what happens to my fringe benefits such as my health insurance, retirement accounts, vacation accrual, etc.?
- Do I have to return to my previous employer, or may I voluntarily terminate my employment to work for a new employer when my physician releases me? What happens to my benefits if this happens?

## Maximum Medical Improvement

*T*here comes a point in every person's recovery which signifies he has reached a plateau. A question frequently asked by patients who are still suffering from the ill effects of their injuries is, "How can I be at a Maximum Medical Improvement when I still have all these problems?" They can require ongoing care, or have severe pain, and yet they are told that there is nothing more that will change their situation. They can have a residual permanent partial or total disability and still be at Maximum Medical Improvement (MMI). They can even find themselves released to return to work for several months or even a year or two before their doctor places them at MMI.

### MMI Is Important

Maximum Medical Improvement (MMI) is also referred to as Medical End Result (MER). Some states use the term Permanent and Stationary (P&S). Which term is used is unimportant, as they are often used interchangeably—sometimes even in the same conversation. (For this book we will use MMI, but you should keep in mind that others may use MER or P&S to refer to the same thing.) MMI is an important point to finally reach in your recovery. It can have significant physical, financial and emotional results for the claimant who has had a long struggle with her recovery and continues to have significant ongoing problems, but is deemed medically stable.

### MMI Does Not Mean You Are Cured

When you reach MMI it simply means that you have reached the point in your illness or injury at which you are not expected to experience any significant improvement or change. This does not mean that all of your problems are cured or resolved. You may still have some serious, permanent problems; for example—you may have terrible chronic pain, blindness or the inability to perform your own care independently. Whatever the symptoms, you will have reached the point at which the physicians say that regardless of your situation, additional treatment is unlikely to produce significant change in your overall end result. You may continue to receive physical therapy, but now it is considered maintenance therapy. You may be using a lot of medications all of the time, but they are not expected to do anything but help you maintain where you are or prevent further complications. Care which you receive from that point forward is considered maintenance care; it is not expected to improve your situation, but neither should your condition worsen.

### Assessing For Determination Of MMI

The physician will not place you at MMI without an adequate assessment of your current condition and treatment plan. You may need to have an Independent Medical Evaluation (IME) or Agreed Medical Examination (AME) to determine if you are at MMI. Regardless of who identifies the term and applies it to your situation, the end result is the same: What you have is what you have. You may need to continue to treat for years, but it will not significantly change the overall picture for you. Some patients may actually return to work—either in a light-duty or full-duty position—and they will not be placed at MMI by their doctors. The opinions about when a person is at MMI can vary from physician to physician.

## Disputing A Determination Of MMI

If you have an IME physician state you are at MMI, yet your own treating physician disagrees, you may be able to buy some additional time with an appeal or dispute. However, you can be sure that if the carrier ordered the IME, and the IME report indicates that you are at MMI, the carrier will do whatever they have to do to ensure your claim is soon closed or denied. If your physician supports you, you may be able to file an appeal with the workers' compensation board representative. However, this must be done immediately, or you may find that you are without your weekly benefits until the dispute is resolved. Most states have firm guidelines outlining any rights you have to appeal certain determinations. If you are able to provide documentation to the state immediately to dispute the claim, you may be able to protect or reinstate your benefits. If you expect to have this type of success with your dispute you will need to be very organized and timely with your argument. You may also request the carrier offer to pay for another opinion or assessment if the determination is in direct contradiction to your treating physician's. This may or may not work to your advantage. You should clarify all of the options with the regulating agency representative and/or your attorney.

Do not waste time trying to call the carrier. The carrier has what they want: A statement which allows them to close or deny your claim. It is up to you to fight the determination if you feel you are not at MMI. But again, remember—just because you continue to have terrible pain or disability, it does not mean that you have not stabilized or reached a plateau. If you can provide documentation which supports there can be an expected change in your condition—either improvement or further deterioration, within a certain period of time given additional treatment—you may be able to successfully argue you have not reached MMI.

## Assessing For Permanent Disability

Once you are at MMI, the carrier may have your physician, the IME physician, or even yet another physician assess for residual permanent partial disability (PPD) or permanent total disability (PTD). If you have reached MMI, you can expect to find documentation somewhere about a permanent partial impairment (PPI) evaluation or determination. When you are given a permanent partial impairment ruling, it simply means that based on a review of you and your past records and treatment, you have some residual disability which is expected to be permanent. The permanent partial impairment rating is usually presented either as a percent of the whole body or the affected body region. When a permanent partial impairment rating is applied, this means you will have some degree of permanent impairment. This impairment can either be a functional impairment, meaning that you have actually lost a percentage of function in the affected area, or the impairment can imply that you have a residual chronic pain syndrome with or without direct involvement or changes in the anatomic structures of the region affected.

## Assigning A Percent Of Disability

When you have a permanent partial impairment evaluation completed, the physician who assigns the degree of impairment usually will use a standardized evaluation tool. Some states have their own evaluation and permanent impairment rating system. In most cases the physician will use the *American Medical Association Guide to the Evaluation of Permanent Impairment* (often referred to simply as the *Guide*). There are currently five editions of the *Guide* to date. Most state regulations will stipulate which edition of the *Guide* must be utilized to assign a degree of permanent partial impairment. As you read through your records it will be important for you to pay attention to which *Guide* was used. The report that identifies your degree of permanent partial impairment should be quite specific and address exactly which section and page the physician referenced to make the determination. If you know your state requires the fifth edition be used and the physician does not specify this in his report, you should request clarification in writing from the physician, with a copy of your request sent to the state regulating agency and the carrier. This can be an important technicality for you to note. The *Guide* changes with each edition and the changes are subtle in some instances. These subtle changes can have significant financial implications for you. When a physician is utilizing the *Guide*, he or she must have participated in an extensive training seminar which outlines specifically how the *Guide* is to be used. The *Guide* is very cumbersome and complicated and can easily be misinterpreted without the proper training.

### Calculating Permanency

Most physicians are well-versed in their knowledge and application of the *Guide*. However, there are physicians who feel they can circumvent the requirements which state they must use a certain edition of it. It is costly for the physician to attend the training and certification for each updated edition of the *Guide*, but it can be much more costly to you as the individual who is the recipient of an improperly calculated permanent impairment rating. In the workers' compensation system, the state may assign a specific dollar amount (or certain number of weeks of temporary total disability) for each percent of permanent partial impairment. For example, if you live in a state where each percent of permanent partial disability equals 5 weeks of temporary total disability payments, if there is a miscalculation of three or four percent, this can substantially reduce the amount of permanent partial disability which you will be awarded. Check with the regulating agency for your individual state's calculations.

### The Amount Of Permanency Awarded

The carrier will be looking for the smallest percent of permanent partial disability to be assigned to your assessment. If you are fortunate enough to live in a state that awards a lump sum payment for a permanent partial disability award, you may actually end up with a little cash in your pocket; or you may receive monthly benefits or ongoing weekly benefits for a period of time. If you feel that the amount of permanency that has been applied to your situation is too small, you should consult with an attorney and arrange to have your own permanent partial impairment evaluation completed. Before you see another physician, you need to clarify what happens if he offers a substantially lower or higher impairment calculation. Many states will take an average of the two amounts while some utilize the lowest percent.

### Your Physician Can Weigh In On Your Permanency Evaluation

When a client has her own physician do a permanent partial impairment evaluation, it is important to remember that whomever you hire to perform the exam must adhere to the same regulations as the carrier's physician and utilize the appropriate *Guide*. The physician should be trained in the appropriate application of the *Guide* and be able to identify what your residual disability is. Do not expect that your physician should or will apply a large degree of permanency just because he is your personal choice to perform the exam. If there is a large discrepancy in the results of the two exams, the state regulations most likely address what will happen in this instance. In some states, the regulations are quite specific and address the issue by requiring that the carrier take an average of the two amounts. In other cases, the state may leave it up to the discretion of the carrier, in which case you will receive the smaller permanency regardless of who assessed it. It is important to clarify with your state agency or attorney what will be the best way for you to proceed. You are not advised to call the carrier to clarify this issue, as they are going to be looking for the least expensive way to finalize your claim. Ethically, they should provide you with the appropriate way to formulate your dispute, but you need to understand that they do not stay in business by paying large sums if they can avoid it.

### After The Final Determination Of Permanency

Once there is a final determination of what your permanency amount will be, you will receive a very complicated form from the carrier and the state which spells out what your permanent impairment percent is and what that means for you. It should state how much the percent is and the dollar amount that this percent represents. This form is usually very complex. There are often many different ways that a claim can be closed or finalized, and this form may have the various options identified on it. Sometimes, your permanent impairment is straightforward; for example, you may receive a percent or two and there is no expectation that you will need additional care in the future. In other situations, you may actually be expected to have a surgical procedure as a direct result of your injury as you age. In this case, it is important to have the correct documentation in your letter of notification about your file closure. If the physicians expect that you will need periodic care in the future that will cause temporary periods of disability, or contribute to an increase in your final disability later on, it is important that this be identified in your letter. If you have any questions at all about this, contact an attorney or the state agency. Your signature is usually required on this form. Make sure you understand everything before you sign.

### The Carrier Is Not Your Advocate

As discussed, your carrier is out to save themselves money. They are in business to make a profit, not to protect your interests.

When Mark received his letter of discontinuance (file closure), Beth—the state agency representative with whom he had been working—noticed the carrier had not addressed the potential need for future care. The carrier had signed a discontinuance that would have completely disallowed any future medical care or disability benefits to be covered under the statement. If Beth had not identified this error, Mark would not be able to file for benefits in the future should the need arise. When Mark spoke to the carrier about his call with Beth, the carrier gave him an entirely different story and went so far as to tell him that Beth was wrong. Further investigation revealed it was indeed the carrier who was in error. Mark's future benefits were protected and the discontinuance was amended with the correct information.

### Requesting A Formal Hearing

Once you have gotten to MMI and you have been assigned a permanent partial impairment evaluation, if you still feel you have been unfairly assessed, you should contact your state agency to request a formal hearing before an Administrative Law Judge. This can be a very stressful and scary position in which to find yourself; it may help you to have an attorney or strong personal advocate available to assist you through the process. If you feel that you deserve more than what is being assessed, you will need to understand what your state's rules are for someone in your position. It is important to remember, though—once you go before the Administrative Law Judge, it is possible (depending on your individual state's rules) that you may actually have your claim denied.

### The Administrative Law Process

The Administrative Law process is a formal legal process which can take place in person or even by an initial telephone conference; but either way, you need to understand how the possible outcomes may affect your claim. If your state representative feels that there is some benefit in a negotiation, she may have you participate in a preliminary conference call with herself and the carrier to try to avoid the formal hearing process. This can be beneficial to you, particularly if you can resolve the conflict without an attorney. Any work which an attorney completes on your behalf—and any fees that he charges—may come directly off the top of any final award or permanency settlement that you receive.

### Changing The Laws

As insurance and workers' compensation rates escalate, many states are amending their rules and laws in an effort to curb costs. In many instances these changes are brought before the legislative branches without the citizens even being aware of what the final outcomes can mean to them, their families and their friends. When the lawmakers are presented with requests for amendments to help reduce the costs of claims, they are often presented with the costs as they relate to the businesses in the state. Lawmakers are influenced by the wishes of their constituents (the people who voted for them), but it is important to realize that the business industry itself is also a constituent. By virtue of its financial strength, businesses have a much louder voice. The lawmakers may make it seem like the changes are for the overall good of the people, but the question is, for *which* people are they best? If you are injured and already in the system prior to new amendments, it is likely that you will continue on in the system under the rules that were in place at the time of your injury. (This is known as being "grandfathered" in.) If you sustain a future injury, you may find that what happened previously—to a coworker or friend, or even yourself—no longer applies, because of changes to the laws.

### Keep Your Binder For The Future

If you have reached an end to your claim (you are at MMI and have received your permanent impairment award), do not discard your paperwork. Keep your binder in a safe place. The final discontinuance paperwork may actually stipulate what happens in the future should your claim need to be reopened. If the paperwork states that you have the right to be covered for future medical care, do not be fooled into thinking the process will be a simple one when it comes time to reopen the claim—especially if some time has passed. That process can be a very difficult battle. The documentation provided by your physicians, and the wording in that documentation, may be the keys to acceptance or denial of the liability for the claim in the future. The state will have specific rules regarding how documentation supports whether the claim is for a new injury or an exacerbation of the old injury. This documentation will be crucial to the determination of your benefits. You can expect that the process to reinstate your benefits can be a long and tedious battle if the documentation is not clear. If you go down this road again, you will need to follow all of the previously outlined steps to have a successful resolution the second time around.

### The Permanency Settlement Can Affect Other Benefits

One final note about any permanency you may receive: If you have been successfully awarded a long-term disability benefit award, such as Social Security Disability, it is important to understand how a lump sum or large financial award for permanency will affect your monthly disability benefits. If you do not notify the Social Security Administration or the Medicaid system about your award, you might face charges of insurance fraud. You will need to contact the other agencies with which you are dealing to discuss how the award will impact any other benefits which you receive.

### The Actual Award May Be Substantially Less

If you are not a claimant in the workers' compensation system and you are at MMI and have been assigned a permanent impairment rating, and you anticipate receiving a settlement from a suit or claim against another party, you will need to clarify whether or not your settlement may be reduced. For example, if you have an automobile liability claim, and are currently collecting workers' compensation benefits for the same accident, it is possible that should you successfully settle against the automobile liability carrier, your workers' compensation carrier will subrogate (take back any money that they paid) against the award which you receive.

Consider a case where you were driving a vehicle for work. You are involved in a motor vehicle accident and the other driver is to blame. You may find that you are given workers' compensation benefits for your temporary total disability until you are able to return to work. While you are out of work you need to have surgery and some rehabilitation as well as medical equipment and medications. Your workers' compensation, or possibly your health insurance, may cover some of these bills. In the meantime, you have also hired an attorney to file a suit against the other driver. Assume you are successful in your suit against the other driver and are awarded a large sum of money. As discussed in a previous chapter, it is important to understand you may not see the entire amount of this award. The insurance that paid your medical bills and perhaps covered your weekly temporary total disability payments may subrogate (take back) the amount of money they paid out on your behalf. Next, your attorney will collect his fee, including expenses. You will end up with what is left. Unfortunately, this may be a vastly different amount than what you were awarded from the suit.

The settlement of the suit may also have a stipulation that some or all of the funds go into a trust, structured settlement, or (MSA) which restricts your access to the settlement money. This can all be very confusing, and you may need to have your attorney clarify it for you. It sounds great to think that you might get an award of a quarter of a million dollars if another party is found liable; however, if there has been a similar amount paid out on your behalf by another carrier, and your attorney takes his portion, you could conceivably end up with very little in the end. Make sure you understand what the agreement means and how the funds will be disbursed.

## Things To Remember

- MMI indicates a plateau in your condition.
- Treatment may continue beyond the determination of MMI, but does not mean you can expect your condition to change or improve.
- You can dispute the determination of MMI.
- You may have a residual permanent partial or total disability.
- The carrier is not your advocate and will search for a way to reduce the amount of any settlement you receive.
- You may need to request an Administrative Law hearing to resolve discrepancies or issues not addressed.
- Maintain your file (binder) indefinitely in case of future problems or need for treatment.
- If the carrier subrogates, the settlement you actually receive may be significantly less than you anticipate.

## Questions You Need To Ask

- What does it mean if I am at MMI (Maximum Medical Improvement) or MER (Medical End Result)?
- How will the determination of MMI or MER affect my benefits?
- What if I disagree with the determination?
- How can I dispute the determination?
- What happens to my benefits if I appeal a determination of MMI?
- Who can determine that I have reached MMI?
- If the IME reports I am at MMI, but my physician disagrees, how will this affect my claim, and what can I do to protect my interests?
- What if the carrier is not acting appropriately—who at the regulating agency will be able to advocate for me? Do I need a lawyer?
- Have I obtained copies of my entire record for this claim from each of my providers, the carrier and the case managers? Do these records support that I am at MMI?
- If I am at MMI, but may need future medical care, how will I have my claim reopened and the care covered?
- What about reimbursement for lost wages if I am unable to work, should the condition worsen or recur?

# 15

## *Friends, Family, Community*

Who are your real friends? This should be an easy question to answer, but in fact it often is not. Until you face the challenges of an injury or illness, you may not discover who your real friends are. Not until you look to your family, friends, coworkers or healthcare team might you find out upon whom you can and cannot count. Most people are blessed with a wide network of support. For many, though, injury and illness can bring out the worst in everyone. It is a time when you learn upon whom you can trust and rely.

### Strength From Family

Unfortunately for some, their network of support is like a large-weave net: full of holes and not the least bit supportive. Families can be our greatest source of strength and support. They may offer love and attention and help us meet all of our needs. On the other hand, they may be elusive. If you have a family that smothers you with affection, relish it. Some of the most frustrating challenges in caring for patients can come when they are all but abandoned by their families. Others have small or non-existent families. And still others come from family environments which are so dysfunctional that when help is offered, it only serves to complicate the patient's recovery.

### Families Need Limits

If you belong to a doting, supportive family, one of the greatest challenges will be to set limits on the support you receive. As you recover you may find yourself overwhelmed with family visitors and advice. They mean well, but sometimes the sheer number of them is exhausting. You will need to find a way to thank them for their support, while at the same time ask them to be just a bit less supportive. It is difficult for some families to know when enough is enough, and it can be tricky to be able to express this without making everyone feel bad. This is a good time to have one person who oversees the masses and acts as your spokesperson and advocate.

### Restricting Visitors

It can be amazing to see how unaware and inconsiderate others can be. The last thing you need to worry about when you are trying to recover from an injury or illness is offending someone. This is your time to heal. This can be especially troublesome if you are hospitalized for a prolonged period of time. It can be draining on the hospitalized patient to have a steady stream of visitors. It can also make it difficult for the staff to manage the care that needs to be given. This is why visitation hours are so restricted.

You will also need to appoint a single representative to meet with your physician. Physicians have limited amounts of time, so it will be even more important for you to have a spokesperson who can meet with the physicians. It is nearly impossible for a physician to meet with a family of ten or twenty members for every patient he has in the hospital every day. He would never be able to accomplish any work. Occasional family meetings with the staff can work well, but it is not feasible to have a group session every day or every shift. Unless there is some critical change in your condition, your family can expect to have a daily update through the physician or his assistant. The nursing staff is more accessible, but will also have to limit the number of family members with whom they meet. If you are planning an elective hospitalization, it would be wise to appoint a single family member to be the liaison between the staff, the rest of the family and yourself.

## Friendships May Change

Friends can be like family members in time of need. They can be either overwhelmingly supportive, or they run in the opposite direction. You will find out in very short order who your friends are when you develop an illness or sustain an injury. If your injury or illness goes on for a long time, it is not uncommon for the nature of your friendships to change. The bonds either grow stronger or they break apart forever. Friends are not like our family. They do not have genetic ties that bind. They are the reflections of our lives, our joys and our sorrows. If our friends have struggles in their own lives, they may not be able to handle the additional challenges, burdens and sorrows our situation poses. Our friends may feel it is okay to back away from the relationship as our situation reminds them of their own frailties. Our friends may assume our families will be our support, which makes them feel that their absence will not be noticed.

It can be hard for the sick or injured person to reach out to friends. Pride may prevent you from reaching out to them. You may feel abandoned and resentful. You may regret you are not able to participate in the relationship as you once did. Regardless, this is the time when you may need your friends the most. The best you can hope for is that your true friends will stick by you. Those that turn their backs in your time of need were not really your friends. This loss may compound your feelings of sadness and isolation as you try to heal. If you find yourself abandoned and alone, it is important you reach out to those few that are standing by. Isolation and sadness can lead to depression and feelings of worthlessness. If you feel this is happening, you need to let your physician know. Depression can have serious negative effects on the healing process.

## Work Relationships Change

Our friends and families are not the only people who can abandon us in our troubled times. It is not uncommon for work relationships to deteriorate, especially if the relationship was crumbling prior to the accident or illness. Supervisors can see your time away from work as just one more hole in the schedule, failing to see the human in need. Coworkers may have been overworked before you left on disability, and now that you are out on leave and there is no temporary relief, they may feel angry and resentful. They resent they have to do additional work without the benefit of additional pay. Some will even express they have doubts about your illness or injury. You may find that those who lack compassion and voice the negative remarks are usually the ones, who—if given the opportunity—would take advantage of the company. They are usually tired, overworked, underpaid, and feeling less than appreciated. They are often the workers who are the least productive. They feel that by being out of work, regardless of your injury and suffering, you are somehow getting something for nothing. They may even secretly wish it were them.

## Resentment Among Coworkers

Resentment may continue at the time you return to work. It is not uncommon for people who return from a period of disability to be faced with the nastiness of bitter coworkers. Oftentimes when patients are released to return to light-duty positions to transition back to work, they will hear snide comments and resentful remarks from their coworkers. If this is something you experience, it is important you speak to your supervisor or HR representative about the problem. You have the right to work in an environment which is supportive and productive. You do not have to be subject to the conditions of a hostile work environment.

## Professionals Without Compassion

One final place where you may be surprised by the lack of support is in the medical community. Most physicians, nurses and healthcare providers have an abundance of compassion. There are others without the slightest bit of compassion, who display a most profound lack of caring or concern. Perhaps it is because they are tired of hearing the same story over and over. Or, perhaps they were always resentful and mean-spirited. Although they are part of a small minority, some of the most uncaring, unfeeling people you may meet are in the medical profession. Perhaps they have never experienced an illness or injury, or perhaps they do not feel the physical level of pain and discomfort that some people do. Whatever the reason, it can be terribly disheartening to have the one group to which you look for support treat you with disrespect if you complain of pain—especially chronic pain. If you find yourself the object of this type of humiliation, you should immediately remove yourself from the situation. If it is physically impossible to do, then you must call for a supervisor and report the offense. If a professional acts in an unprofessional manner and you feel your basic human rights have been violated, you or your representative should contact your state's agency responsible for professional licensure and conduct. It is inexcusable that you should ever feel your complaints, your illness or your injury are ridiculed and not taken seriously.

When you visit each medical facility and provider, the Patient's Bill of Rights will usually be on display. These are your rights and responsibilities as a patient. If you feel your care does not meet these standards, it must be reported. You can be sure—if it has happened to you, it most likely has happened to others.

### Other Places For Support

Solitude can sometimes be a tremendous blessing. But for those who feel the despair of being abandoned and alone without any source of support, there are resources. You can contact your local Human Services Agency, your church or community service outreach agency. Many regions have offices established specifically to assist and advocate for individuals with disabilities. Find a professional; speak to your physician, your carrier or a friend or family member to help you find assistance in coping with the emptiness and hopelessness. Regardless of whom you choose, do not suffer your situation alone.

### Talking To Family And Friends

When you are injured or become ill, you will eventually share information about your condition with your family and maybe your friends. Not everyone feels comfortable sharing what might be bad news with their family and friends, but eventually the news will come out. There is no right or wrong way to handle sharing this information. As with anything else, you need to be honest. You might not need to go into every single detail, but offer honest, concise information. This will prevent misunderstandings. It will help people understand what is happening and maybe help them to be supportive of you. If you are honest and let people know what is going on with you, you will be less likely to be looked upon with suspicion or pity.

Not everyone will be supportive, but if you have been honest with them, you leave the door open for them to process the information and offer help if they feel they can. When you talk with your coworkers, unless they are close friends, you might want to be a little less open. Too much information in the workplace among coworkers can generate all sorts of problems. Coworkers will either be very supportive, or you may be faced with resentment and distrust.

Provide information to your supervisor or Human Resource manager per your company policies to make sure you do not jeopardize your work-related claim. If this is not work-related but you feel that you want to share the information about your illness or injury, you may encounter similar negativity. You might be very surprised to find out who is supportive and who is not in the workplace. Be honest with your information, but do not offer more information than you want spread throughout the company. Any information you share is likely to be shared with everyone. You might be the talk of the company, but the story may be very different as it is passed from one coworker to the next. This is especially true if you have had any problems on a personal level with any of your coworkers.

When Lynn injured her back, she expected her coworkers—a large group of nurses—would be supportive. Surely they would understand what she had experienced. When Mary injured her knee and had an arthroscopy and meniscectomy, she also hoped her coworkers would be supportive, as they were this same group of nurses. As it turned out, these nurses as a group were overworked, understaffed and underpaid for their expertise. Having two injured coworkers contributed even more to their workloads and the requirements for them to fill in with overtime and come in on their off days. Instead of being supportive to the two injured women, they were a nasty group who made snide remarks, even commenting that both of them were somehow enjoying their poor health because it gave them a break from having to do "real work." This was very evident when both women were working in a light-duty capacity for the department. Lynn and Mary were treated like outcasts and stories were spread about the "real reasons" the women were not working on the unit.

Both eventually returned to full duty, but not without the scars and underlying hurt and disappointment caused by their coworkers. Both women had been as honest as they could. They provided exquisite detail to their friends at work, but neither was prepared for the backlash that came from being injured. Each time they provided updated information after their appointments, it seemed to aggravate their friends and coworkers even more. They were surprised to find a group of people who could offer such support, understanding and skilled care to their patients could be so cold, calculating and unsupportive of them in their time of need. The thing to remember is that this can pertain to any coworkers in any profession.

When you share your information with your family and friends, be cautious as well. Your family and friends might react like your coworkers, but for different reasons. They might worry about losing you because they love you as a valued family member or friend; or they may resent the fact that your illness or injury has changed the dynamics of your relationship. They might have always been able to lean on you for support and now they might be called on to provide support they do not feel capable of or willing to offer.

## The Flip Side Of The Coin

If you are on the other side of the relationship, you may have just as many obstacles. If you are the coworker, family member or friend, do not try to force things. Let your ailing friend or family member know you are there to help him if you can and if he wants it from you. It can be very difficult for people to ask for help. Do not assume that because someone has not directly asked for your help that he does not need or want it. You might try to suggest that you would like to do some errands for him or help him get to his appointments. Maybe bringing by a snack or meal would be helpful. But do not do this and expect some great reward. Some people are so overwhelmed with their illness or injury that they forget to say thank you.

Do not assume if information is given to you by your friend or coworker that he wants you to announce the information to the rest of the world. Before you share whatever information has been given to you, check with the person to see if this is okay. Do not assume that because he told you about his illness or injury he would feel comfortable with the rest of the company, neighborhood or even family knowing. Ask if he needs anything, and be prepared to follow through. Do not make empty promises and let down the patient. If you say you can drive him to an appointment or run an errand, be true to your word. You likely appreciate his honesty and he will appreciate yours as well.

## *Things To Remember*

- A time of need can let you know who your real friends are.
- Families can be supportive; but without limits, they may hinder your recovery.
- Too many visitors can impede your recovery and hinder the care provided by the professionals.
- Friendships, work relationships and family dynamics can change.
- Coworkers can be resentful.
- Not everyone will be compassionate.

- There are many places for support.
- Do not ignore feelings of emptiness, hopelessness or despair.

## *Questions You Need To Ask*

- On whom can I truly count for support, understanding and guidance?
- Have I appointed a family spokesperson or advocate?
- If I have problems at work with coworkers, how will my employer manage the situation?
- Am I physically and mentally capable of returning to my former employer or position?
- Does my family know and accept their boundaries, or do I need someone to intervene on my behalf?
- If I feel that my providers lack compassion and caring, is there an advocate who will intervene to address the situation?
- Have I realistically faced the changes in myself, my relationships and possible future plans as affected by my recent illness or injury?

# 16

## *Your New Self*

*F*inally, you have reached the point where you no longer are running to appointments all of the time. You have reached MMI and are now trying to readjust to your life with or without permanent residual disabilities. Making the transition physically and mentally can be a challenge. Even if you feel great, you have still experienced a traumatic event which will make you stronger, or—for some—erode what little self-confidence you had.

### Change Can Be Stressful

As you will undoubtedly come to realize, change can have a very positive or negative effect on your life. But ultimately it is a desire to survive which will impact your ability to adapt to the change. That being said, it is important to understand the final change can—and most likely will—be stressful to you, your family and your friends. Change is without a doubt stressful whether it is something we eagerly choose for ourselves, or something which has been forced upon us. In the end, it is our very human nature which will allow us to adapt and appreciate the new direction life takes us. As you settle into your new routine, you will adapt to the changes by going through several steps which are quite similar to those experienced by people who have had a loss in their life.

### Change Produces Anxiety

Any change, positive or negative, will produce a certain amount of anxiety. If you can be aware of this before it happens, and as it happens, it can help you make the transition without imposing more stress on yourself. As you went through the process from injury to recovery, you experienced not only physical but emotional stress. Adapting to those stressors helped you to finally progress to where you are today. It can be anxiety-provoking to have to adapt again.

### You Cannot Always Control Change

When we adapt to stress we pass through many stages, but one of the most beneficial tools is to accept that some of the changes are beyond our control. There are some changes which you can control. It is important and positive to accept that you made it through these changes with the knowledge and resources available to you at that time. It is easy to second-guess everything after it has happened. The best you can hope for is that you do not allow yourself to be regretful and take on additional stress, guilt or self-loathing. They say hindsight is 20/20, or perfect. Every time we utter the phrase "I wish I had…" or "I should have…" we contribute to our guilt and stress. We can make ourselves sick with regret. There comes a time when acceptance of the situation is integral to healing and survival.

### We Cannot Control Others

Earlier, we discussed taking control. This is the time when it is crucial not to lose that control. You cannot control the thoughts, action and speech of others, but you *can* take control of how you respond. When you are questioned or challenged—and inevitably, you will be—you will need to pull back and stand firm. Let others have their say, but know for yourself that whatever you did, you did what you thought was best for you at the time.

## Trust In Yourself

Friends and especially family will have the most to offer. You may find it quite amazing that the people who sat on the sidelines and may have offered help or those who withheld their help and support will be the loudest critics you might face. Stand your ground and do not give in to the criticism and disapproving remarks. If you have gotten to this point, be sure of yourself and trust that you have the strength and the ability to survive the final changes you must face.

## Acknowledge The Change Around You

Your first step is to identify the change. The change related to an illness or injury may be quite obvious, or it may be so subtle that only you know it exists. Some injuries and illnesses leave obvious disfigurements and deformities, while others leave behind an invisible, silent path of chronic pain and suffering. Prior to the injury you may have had an active, enjoyable existence free of any restrictions. You were social and outgoing. Now you are limited by pain or disability and are forced to play a different role with your family, friends and community. You may be forced to adapt to whatever the change is. You may have to learn to live with your restrictions and adapt your life around your limitations and changed abilities.

## Define "It"

At some point in your recovery or rehabilitation, you will invariably hear the words *"You are just going to have to learn to live with it."* And truth be told, you may very well have to. However, before you blindly accept this adage as the way your life will be, demand an explanation of what *"it"* is. A person is better able to adapt and cope with what they know to be a firm fact, rather than a vague concept. Nothing is more infuriating or disheartening than to hear a provider tell a patient they must *"learn to live with it."* As a patient you have the right to know what "it" is and with what, exactly, you are expected to "learn to live." Once you know what "it" is, do some research and learn all you can, so that *you* control *it,* and *it* does not control *you.*

Stephan continued to have severe pain in his back after a nasty lumbar vertebral fracture. He had multiple tests and procedures over the two years since his injury. He continued to have a lot of pain that the doctors could not explain. Over and over he complained and requested several consults, hoping to find an answer. Each doctor with whom he met reviewed his file and examined him and his films. Each one told him the same thing: "You are just going to have to learn to live with it." Stephan was near the end of his rope because he was used to being healthy and active. He had never been sick and he had never needed anything to help him manage any pain he had before his injury.

Finally, he found a physician he could trust. He asked Dr. Martin to explain to him what it was with which he must learn to live. Finally, Dr. Martin told him he had myofascial pain syndrome. At first Stephan thought this was Dr. Martin's polite way to tell him that he was a little crazy and that there was nothing really wrong. Dr. Martin gave him some literature to read and referred him to a pain management specialist. Stephan reviewed the information that he had been given and did some research on his own— and found out there was a physical explanation for his pain. He found out there were actual physiological changes at the cellular level that caused small areas of muscle spasms around some of the nerves in his lower back. Stephan met with the pain management doctor and was given a new treatment plan. Armed with the treatment plan, a specific diagnosis and the ability to research ways to take care of himself, Stephan was able to "live with it." He had finally defined what "it" was. He was able to take control over his situation and become an active participant in his care. Stephan still has occasional episodes where the pain intensifies and hinders some of his activities, but he has learned how to make some adaptations in his life. He is no longer living in the dark as a dependent patient. He is able to be independent and maintain control over his situation. He knows when to call his doctor and when to use some of his self-care techniques.

## Adapting To The Changes

As you begin to formulate a way to live with the changes, you may actually subconsciously or consciously deny the change exists. You may try to perform outside of your restrictions. You may try to forgo the ongoing work or exercise adaptations which allow you to regain your independence. You may even try to stop some medications or perform activities which are dangerous and may even harm you further. But as you forge ahead with your denial firmly intact, the setbacks and exacerbations may serve to return you to the necessary treatment or restrictions. It may help you to finally move to the next step of learning: eventually accepting and adapting to the changes which are now part of your life.

## Grieving For What Once Was

As you deny anything has changed, and as you see the results it can produce, unless you are impaired emotionally and mentally, you will inevitably move towards accepting change. You will grieve what you have lost. You will see sorrow and grief can help you face your changes and move you to the final stages of your healing process. These changes that you grieve may be obvious physical losses. They may be your inability to process and think as you once did. The change may be an outward change in the roles you have with your family, friends and coworkers and community as a whole. It is at this stage of learning to accept change and its impact on our life that we may become bogged down in anxiety and depression. It is at this time you might feel the hopelessness of the situation. You are able to grieve the change, but instead of moving on from your grief, you become stuck. You may have felt the undercurrent of the depression and anxiety earlier, but it may not surface as an obvious component of your reality until you have gone through the other processes and have come to this part of your recovery. Now the final reality of what you have and where you are can stop you cold in your tracks.

## Facing The Crossroads

It can be quite numbing to come face-to-face with the crossroads of your change. The strongest among us can experience a depression to depths which create a feeling of despair and hopelessness. This is the juncture at which it is vital to re-involve the members of your healthcare team. If you feel this is something which you can move through alone, then try to push onward. But if you feel immobilized by the apprehension and hopelessness your new life presents, you must seek professional help. When you try to ignore a true depression and pretend it does not exist, you may have to face it when you are least expecting it to resurface. There is no shame in asking for help to cope with the changes in your life. There is more shame in denying yourself the help you need. If you are concerned about the cost or the time, this may be something to address with your carrier and state agency representative. If your doctor can show your emotional problems are related to your injury or illness, you may be entitled to some psychological care to help you readjust to your situation. Do not let those details stand in the way of your success.

## It's Okay To Grieve

It is expected that you will grieve the changes you are facing. You cannot skip over any step of the process. To try to deny or ignore the feelings which you have will only slow down the success of your recovery. Grieving is a complex process. It presents itself in as many ways as there are people. If you were to ask a hundred people how they grieve, you would have a hundred different responses. There is no correct process and there is no wrong way to grieve. It becomes wrong when you try to deny yourself the experience. Most important for you to remember is that this is an okay feeling for you to have. It becomes not okay when it becomes so deep your very existence is threatened.

## You Cannot Grieve Forever

Although it is expected you will grieve, it is not expected you will do so deeply and forever. If you seek help to move through the process, it will allow you to identify the strengths and abilities in yourself which you did not know existed. When you seek help from a professional, do not expect he will fix the problem. He can guide you through it and he will help you find your own abilities to fix the problem. You will learn what to do to cope. You can seek help from the members of your healthcare team, from a counselor or even a religious leader. There is no best resource for this help. We all respond differently to the various practitioners. It does not matter *who* helps you, but rather that you get the help you need.

### Coming To Terms With Reality

Once you have gone through the steps, you will move to the final stage which allows you to accept your changes. This does not mean you will always be happy with your situation, but it is the point at which you can come to terms with the reality of your circumstances. You will be able to constructively make and accept the changes which will allow you to resume your life. This is the point at which you can realistically see the bad points and the good points. Your situation is different than before. It is here that you can decide to take the control back. You may still have your restrictions, but instead of letting them control you, you learn to control them and your surroundings in a way which is acceptable to you.

### Break Free Of The Label, *"Patient"*

To accept your new-found place in life, with the good and the bad, can be a comforting experience. This can be both liberating and exhilarating, especially if you learn that even with your changes you can find some sense of life and independence. You have endured the troubles your injury or illness forced on you. You have faced the physical challenges. Now you can focus on controlling your destiny. You will need to learn to take advantage of the resources available to you. Your focus can be on the future and with a renewed sense of control you can break free of the label of "patient" or "claimant." It is very liberating to stop referring to yourself as a patient. Before your illness or injury, you probably did not refer to yourself as a "well person" or a "non-patient." Regardless of what residual disabilities you have left, you are no longer a patient. A patient is someone who is in need of care, attention and intervention. You may need care, attention and intervention, but not for the same reasons as when you first were injured or became ill.

### Reclaim Your Control

You are encouraged to accept your place in your process. Work within your means and accept your changes as part of who you are. If you are honest with yourself you may actually find you were not all that perfect prior to your injury or illness. You may find you have a new humility and respect for life which was lacking previously. You will need to take your control back. If you continue to hand over the control of your life to others, you will remain a bitter, resentful, dissatisfied person who focuses on the negatives and ignores the fact that you have survived. To spend your time angrily regretting the hand which is dealt to you will only contribute to feelings of emptiness and bitterness.

### Change Is Continuous

Change is an ongoing process. You can choose some changes and other changes are chosen for you. Every day of your life is about change. Never will you have a day that is exactly as the day before. Some change you can recognize and consciously decide to embrace and reconcile. Change that results from an injury or illness may not be a change which you would have chosen, but if you are fortunate enough to have survived, you owe it to yourself to take control of your life. You may need to depend on the assistance of others; but even then, you can express your desires and regain some control. Change forces growth and this growth can force you in new directions which are ultimately more exciting and rewarding than if you had continued in your existence as before.

### The Glass Is Half Full

If you can see change as a positive glass-half-full event in your life, you will be able to make the necessary adaptations to enjoy and savor what self-respect and self-reliance you have left. Those who are chronically disgruntled, glass-half-empty people will suffer and be full of anger and resentment regardless of what life offers. They will always see their position as something to blame on someone else. Every one of us is given a life to live. Regardless of our situation, we do have the ability to decide whether to accept our successes or dwell in our misery. It is easier to play the blame game than to accept our roles in our lives. Many times accidents and events occur which are beyond our control. Many times we make choices which affect the outcomes from those accidents and events. Our residual restrictions and limitations may significantly impact our lives. Our chronic pain or disfigured bodies may challenge us daily. We can either decide to accept the challenge and move forward as best as we can, or we can sit and let our lives pass us by. We are ultimately responsible for ourselves.

### Life Is Your Gift

Finally you will come to the time when you must accept that you have had the injury or illness. You can be like a broken teacup: You can be glued back together and used lovingly for years to come, or you can throw it all away in a fit of anger and rage and regret that what was broken can never be fixed. Your life can be your gift. You can choose to accept the new gifts and find new ways to use them, or you can sit angrily in the corner blaming others for your misfortune. To cherish life and enjoy every minute is more rewarding, even with all the bumps and misfortunes along the way. You can live your life to its fullest or you can wish and hope that things will change—getting older with each day, and not living and feeling the success inside. You must decide to take control of life's unexpected circumstances before they take control of you.

### Things To Remember

- Change can be stressful.
- Some changes are beyond your control.
- We cannot control the actions of others.
- Trust in yourself.
- Define "it" and learn how to live with "it."
- It is okay to grieve your losses and changes.
- You cannot grieve forever.
- Come to accept your reality.
- Break free of the label, "patient."
- Take back control of your life.
- Your life is your gift.

### Questions You Need To Ask

- Do I understand how my condition will change my life in the future?
- Do I understand the changes with which I may have to live?
- How and where can I find help to adjust to the changes imposed by my condition?
- How can I find help to deal with a depression and grief that is overwhelming me and impeding my recovery?
- Will my carrier cover any counseling or therapy that I may need to help me deal with my depression and adjust to the changes in my life as a result of my condition?
- Have my providers adequately defined "it," so when they say I "have to learn to live with it," I can?
- Have I learned how to take control of my life and my condition?

## Appendix A
## *Glossary of Terms*

**ABMS** American Board of Medical Specialty. They can confirm if your physician is certified in a certain specialty.

**Americans with Disabilities Act (ADA)** Enacted by the federal government. It offers a specific list of guidelines which those in the business world must follow to accommodate the needs of individuals with disabilities. Includes guidelines regarding the design of sites to accommodate access by the disabled individual.

**Adjudicate** To settle a claim or case.

**Adjustor** The adjustor of your claim will review and pay the bills according to the rules and regulations of your jurisdiction. The adjustor may pay less than the billed amount if there is a pre-existing fee schedule or other agreement in place.

**American Medical Association (AMA)** A national organization of physicians that writes, creates and lobbies for healthcare policies.

**Ancillary Provider** A provider of any of the following: skilled nursing, home care, outpatient rehabilitation, transportation, and therapy services; also facility-based services such as ambulatory surgery, dialysis, laboratory and diagnostic imaging.

**Anti-fraud** The name for a unit set up by an insurance company to investigate and prevent fraudulent claims.

**Appeal** The procedure in place to have a claim denial reconsidered. Oftentimes the process to file an appeal is involved, but should be pursued if you feel that a claim was denied in error.

**Average Weekly Wage (AWW)** A computation of the amount of money you earn on a weekly basis. Each state may be different. The average may be determined by using a specific number of weeks.

**Benefit** For the purposes of this book, a benefit is something that will be helpful to you in resolving your claim. For example, your weekly indemnity check from workers' compensation may be your benefit. The benefit is a definition of what you will have coming to you to satisfy your claim as you progress through your illness or injury rehabilitation.

**Benefits Administrator** A person who coordinates and maintains the policies under which you will receive your benefits. He is responsible for ensuring that the benefits are utilized appropriately in conjunction with the policies of the company or agency which he represents.

**Board of Professional Conduct** A professional group designed to ensure ethical and professional codes are maintained by its members. For example, a Board of Conduct for physicians ensures that the physicians under its licensing jurisdiction follow and adhere to a specific code of professional and ethical practice.

**Carrier**   The insurance company paying the bills for your illness or injury.

**Center for Disease Control (CDC)**   The lead federal agency for protecting the health and safety of Americans, both at home and abroad. The CDC serves as the national focus for developing and applying disease prevention and control, environmental health, and health promotion and education activities aimed at improving the health of the people of the United States.

**Claim**   The sum of all of the actions and payments surrounding your illness or injury from insurance and/or state agencies.

**Claimant**   The person who files the claim; the ill or injured individual.

**Claims Representative**   The person responsible for managing your claim at the insurance company/carrier.

**Client**   See **claimant**.

**Computerized Axial Tomography Scan (CT Scan)**   A diagnostic technique which offers a three-dimensional image used to diagnose diseases and conditions of the internal body structures.

**Contingency**   Something dependent on a future outcome. If an attorney takes a personal injury client on contingency, he agrees he will not be paid unless there is a successful outcome to the case.

**Cumulative Trauma Syndrome**   Injuries or illness to various body parts which are typically caused by the repetitive use of the particular body part. These are usually seen in the upper extremities but can affect other body areas, depending upon the type of repetitive activity to which it is subjected. Damage to the muscles, bones and cellular structure of the affected region can result.

**Date of Injury**   The date on which you sustained the injury *or* reported the accident or illness. In some instances it may be different than the actual onset of the symptoms.

**Date of Loss**   Similar to **date of injury**, but may specifically be used to represent the date associated with all of the bills from your claim.

**Disability**   A physical or psychological condition that impairs or limits participation in one or more major life activities.

**Doctor**   The person you hire to be your treating physician. (Can refer to a medical doctor, a doctor of osteopathy, etc.)

**Documentation**   All of the written and computerized information surrounding your claim; the written evidence of the events of your claim.

**Durable Medical Equipment (DME)**   Non-disposable medical supplies, such as walkers and wheelchairs.

**Electromyelogram (EMG)**   A test used to trace the nerve pathways and assess their functions. Can be used to determine if there is nerve damage, and assist in identifying the location of the origin of the problem.

**Employee**   A person who works for another person or group of persons in return for financial compensation.

**Employer**   The person or group who hires, pays and supervises an employee.

**Entitlement**   Something which is owed or expected. This may refer to benefits owed to you as a result of a government regulation. For example, some states mandate that after a period of time, an injured worker may be entitled to have an evaluation to determine if they qualify for vocational rehabilitation benefits.

**Ergonomics**   The science of equipment design and workplace planning, used to reduce the injuries caused by improper and unsafe posture/positioning when performing repetitive and routine activities.

**Fee Schedule**   A set of agreed-upon fees that will be paid for certain procedures and diagnoses.

**Fee-For-Service**   Refers to an amount that will be paid for a service without negotiation of the price.

**Functional Capacity Evaluation (FCE)**   An objective assessment of the injured or ill person's physical capacity either as it relates to the duties of her current job, or for the assessment of her abilities in a new job. It will define the level of activity and physical functioning of the individual.

**Human Resources (HR) Representative**   Oversees the management and implementation of the policies and procedures to be followed by employees of the organization.

**Indemnity**   A monetary benefit that is paid when certain conditions are met. An indemnity benefit does not necessarily pay the actual costs. Sometimes weekly workers' compensation payments are referred to as indemnity benefits.

**Independent Medical Examination (IME)**   An examination performed by a physician who is not your treating physician or provider. It is usually used to establish an objective observation about the current assessment and treatment plan of the patient. It can be used to help make a determination about the causality or relationship of symptoms as they relate to an injury or illness.

**Informed Consent**   An agreement to undertake treatment after having been informed of all of the benefits, risks and expected outcomes and results.

**Joint Commission on Accreditation of Healthcare Organizations (JCAHO)**   The main standard-setting and monitoring organization in the health care industry in the United States.

**Jurisdiction**   Legal authority over a certain region or group.

**Light-Duty Work (LDW)**   Work intended to be less physically demanding and stressful than your primary job. It is used primarily in a transitional manner when trying to gradually bring a person back to work after a time out with an illness or injury.

**Long-Term Disability**   A period of impairment and infirmity that lasts beyond a short period of time. In many instances, a long-term period of disability is defined as beginning at 60 days or 6 months.

**Magnetic Resonance Imaging (MRI)**   A diagnostic imaging technique used to assess the structures of the inside of the body.

**Malpractice**   Improper care or treatment of a patient by a physician or healthcare provider.

**Managed Care**   Care which is organized and coordinated by a group; aims to offer quality healthcare while managing costs and eliminating waste.

**Maximum Medical Improvement (MMI)**   The point at which it is determined that additional care and treatment will have minimal impact on the eventual outcome; it can be demonstrated that there is little else to be gained by ongoing acute care. Oftentimes used interchangeably with **Medical End Result**. Frequently it signifies the point at which reimbursement (such as weekly workers' compensation payments) will be terminated.

**Medical Case Management (MCM)**   Refers to the planning and coordination of healthcare services appropriate to the goal of medical rehabilitation. Medical case management may include—but is not limited to—care assessment (including a personal interview with the injured person); assistance in developing, implementing and coordinating a medical care plan between health care providers, the client and his family; and evaluation of treatment results. Medical case management is not the provision of medical care. The goal of medical case management should be to avail the disabled individual of all appropriate treatment options to ensure the client can make informed choices.

**Medical End Result (MER)**   See **Maximum Medical Improvement**.

**Negligence**   Actions which are careless and undertaken without regard for the accepted standards of care.

**National Institute of Health (NIH)**   The steward of medical and behavioral research for the United States. This agency operates under the aegis of the U.S. Department of Health and Human Services.

**Occupational Health**   The practice and coordination of the scope of medicine geared towards occupational health and safety in industry.

**Occupational Safety & Health Association (OSHA)**   The government agency that establishes and enforces protective standards for workplaces, as well as reaches out to employers and employees through technical assistance and consultation programs.

**Out-of-Work (OOW)**   In the workers' compensation system, this refers to the period of time in which an employee is unable to work due to an illness or injury.

**Payee**   The person who receives a payment. In the workers' compensation system, the claimant is the payee.

**Payor**   The person who provides a payment. In the workers' compensation system, the carrier is the payor.

**Permanency**  See **Permanent Partial Impairment Evaluation.**

**Permanent Partial Impairment Evaluation (PPIE)**  An assessment using formalized criteria (such as the *AMA Guides to the Evaluation of Permanent Impairment*) which identifies and measures what percent of the whole person has a residual impairment or disability. It is the point at which the overall condition is unlikely to change regardless of further medical or surgical intervention. A Permanent Partial Impairment Evaluation is completed once the individual has reached **Maximum Medical Improvement** or **Medical End Result.**

**Physiatrist**  A physician who specializes in physical medicine and rehabilitation.

**Primary Physician**  The physician who coordinates and plans your care and any referrals to specialists. This physician should be managing all of the necessary information between your providers to ensure continuity and safety of care.

**Provider**  Anyone who provides care and/or services to ensure adequate healthcare delivery. Examples of providers: Physician, nurse, physical therapist, DME supplier, etc.

**Registered Nurse (RN)**  A licensed nursing professional charged with the duties of assessing, planning, implementing and evaluation of care for the ill or injured person.

**Repetitive Stress Injury (RSI)**  See **Cumulative Trauma Syndrome.**

**Risk Management**  The process utilized by healthcare providers to assess and control risks that can result in monetary loss.

**Self-Insured**  Term used to describe a company that insures themselves without hiring an outside insurance agency. Typically, a specific amount of money which is projected to cover anticipated costs is set aside.

**Short-Term Disability**  A brief period of disability, oftentimes less than 60 days.

**State Regulating Agency**  The agency appointed by the states to develop, evaluate and enforce the rules and regulations for various services in the state. For example, workers' compensation may be regulated by the state's Department of Labor or a separate workers' compensation division.

**Subrogation**  The substitution of one creditor for another. If one insurer has paid on a claim, and there is available money or another party who is found responsible, the insurer may have the right to take money to satisfy the amount they paid. For example, if there is a car accident and the car insurance pays the medical bills, but then the injured person collects a sum of money in a suit related to the accident, the car insurance may subrogate the funds they paid. This may also happen in third-party-actions or personal injury lawsuits.

**Symptom**  A sign of a problem which may confirm the existence of a disease or injury.

**Third-Party Administrator (TPA)**  An administering agent or company who manages the actual payment and adjudication of claims for another entity or company.

**Transitional Duty**   Work which is intended to offer a bridge between the period of disability and return to full duty.

**Vendor**   A company or person who sells/provides a service or product.

**Vocational Rehabilitation (Voc Rehab)**   The coordination of a comprehensive vocational assessment, determination of transferable skills, functional capacity evaluation, career counseling and job-search assistance.

**Workers' Compensation**   Insurance provided by an employer to cover employee costs associated with a work-related illness or injury when the individual is unable to perform the usual and customary duties of his occupation. Benefits may also include compensation on a scheduled basis to cover lost wages until the individual is able to return to work.

## Appendix B – Reference Forms

### Patient Worksheet
*Be sure to copy each form before you complete it.*
Complete this and insert into your permanent file. Bring it with you to each appointment.

| | |
|---|---|
| Name | |
| Address | |
| | |
| Phone | |
| Emergency Contact & Phone | |
| Date of Birth | |
| Social Security Number | |
| Date of Injury/Illness | |
| Date Reported | |
| Reported To | |
| Related to Work? | Yes          No |
| Related to Auto? | Yes          No |
| | Attach a copy of your written report to this form. |

Employment Information

| | |
|---|---|
| Employer | |
| Address | |
| | |
| Phone and Fax | |
| Contact | |
| Supervisor | |
| Job Title | |
| Position | Full Time          Part Time          Temporary |
| Last Day of Work | |
| Date Returned | |

Health Insurance Information

| | |
|---|---|
| Company Name | |
| Address | |
| | |
| Phone and Fax | |
| Adjustor's Name | |
| ID# | |
| Claim # | |
| Workers' Comp # | |

State-Federal Regulating Agency

| Agency Name | |
|---|---|
| Case Worker | |
| Address | |
| | |
| Phone and Fax | |
| Case # | |

Attorney

| Name | |
|---|---|
| Address | |
| | |
| Phone and Fax | |
| Assistant | |

Primary Care Physician

| Name | |
|---|---|
| Address | |
| | |
| Phone and Fax | |
| Assistant | |

Physician

| Name | |
|---|---|
| Address | |
| | |
| Phone and Fax | |
| Assistant | |
| Specialty | |
| Dates of Treatment | |

Physician

| Name | |
|---|---|
| Address | |
| | |
| Phone and Fax | |
| Assistant | |
| Specialty | |
| Dates of Treatment | |

Physician

| Name | |
|---|---|
| Address | |
| | |
| Phone and Fax | |
| Assistant | |
| Specialty | |
| Dates of Treatment | |

Physician

| Name | |
|---|---|
| Address | |
| | |
| Phone and Fax | |
| Assistant | |
| Specialty | |
| Dates of Treatment | |

Physician

| Name | |
|---|---|
| Address | |
| | |
| Phone and Fax | |
| Assistant | |
| Specialty | |
| Dates of Treatment | |

Physical Therapy

| Name | |
|---|---|
| Address | |
| | |
| Phone and Fax | |
| Assistant | |

Occupational Therapy

| Name | |
|---|---|
| Address | |
| | |
| Phone and Fax | |
| Assistant | |

Other Therapy

| Name | |
|---|---|
| Address | |
| | |
| Phone and Fax | |
| Assistant | |

Pharmacy

| Name | |
|---|---|
| Address | |
| | |
| Phone and Fax | |
| Pharmacist | |

Pharmacy

| Name | |
|---|---|
| Address | |
| | |
| Phone and Fax | |
| Pharmacist | |

Medical Case Manager

| Name | |
|---|---|
| Address | |
| | |
| Phone and Fax | |

Vocational Case Manager

| Name | |
|---|---|
| Address | |
| | |
| Phone and Fax | |

Medical Supply Vendor

| Name | |
|---|---|
| Address | |
| | |
| Phone and Fax | |
| Equipment Supplied | |

Medical Supply Vendor

| Name | |
|---|---|
| Address | |
| | |
| Phone and Fax | |
| Equipment Supplied | |

Hospital

| Name | |
|---|---|
| Address | |
| | |
| Phone and Fax | |
| Dates of Admission | |

Hospital

| Name | |
|---|---|
| Address | |
| | |
| Phone and Fax | |
| Dates of Admission | |

Diagnosis for this injury or illness

| |
|---|
| |
| |
| |
| |
| |

Surgeries related to this illness or injury

| Description | Date |
|---|---|
| | |
| | |
| | |
| | |
| | |

Tests and treatments you have had for this problem

| Description | Date |
|---|---|
| | |
| | |
| | |
| | |
| | |

Medications you are taking
(Include prescription and over-the-counter preparations as well as any herbal therapies.)

| Name | Dose | Frequency | Reason |
|---|---|---|---|
| | | | |
| | | | |
| | | | |
| | | | |
| | | | |
| | | | |
| | | | |
| | | | |
| | | | |

Allergies
(Include all medicines, food and environmental allergies.)

|  |
| --- |
|  |
|  |
|  |
|  |
|  |

Past medical history
(List any prior accidents, illnesses or medical conditions for which you have been treated by a physician.)

| Description | Date |
| --- | --- |
|  |  |
|  |  |
|  |  |
|  |  |
|  |  |
|  |  |
|  |  |
|  |  |
|  |  |
|  |  |

Symptoms of your current injury or illness
(Make a note of when they first appeared.)

| Symptoms | Date |
| --- | --- |
|  |  |
|  |  |
|  |  |
|  |  |
|  |  |
|  |  |
|  |  |
|  |  |
|  |  |
|  |  |

List remedies which have helped your condition.

|  |
| --- |
|  |
|  |
|  |
|  |
|  |

List remedies which have worsened your condition.

|  |
| --- |
|  |
|  |
|  |
|  |
|  |

Make sure to note any additional information you feel is pertinent to this claim.

## Communications Log
*Be sure to copy each form before you complete it.*
(Fill out with each communication you complete. Insert into your permanent file.)

| Contact | Date/Time | Method | Contact Reason |
|---------|-----------|--------|----------------|
|         |           |        |                |
|         |           |        |                |
|         |           |        |                |
|         |           |        |                |
|         |           |        |                |
|         |           |        |                |
|         |           |        |                |
|         |           |        |                |
|         |           |        |                |
|         |           |        |                |
|         |           |        |                |
|         |           |        |                |
|         |           |        |                |
|         |           |        |                |
|         |           |        |                |
|         |           |        |                |
|         |           |        |                |
|         |           |        |                |
|         |           |        |                |
|         |           |        |                |
|         |           |        |                |
|         |           |        |                |
|         |           |        |                |
|         |           |        |                |
|         |           |        |                |
|         |           |        |                |
|         |           |        |                |
|         |           |        |                |
|         |           |        |                |
|         |           |        |                |
|         |           |        |                |
|         |           |        |                |
|         |           |        |                |
|         |           |        |                |
|         |           |        |                |
|         |           |        |                |
|         |           |        |                |
|         |           |        |                |
|         |           |        |                |
|         |           |        |                |

## Questions For Your Doctor
*Be sure to copy each form before you complete it.*
(List questions to be discussed at your next appointment, answers to your questions
and treatment plan. Keep a running log. Insert into your permanent file after each physician visit.)

| Date | Questions/Concerns | Doctor's Answers/Plan |
|------|--------------------|-----------------------|
|      |                    |                       |
|      |                    |                       |
|      |                    |                       |
|      |                    |                       |
|      |                    |                       |
|      |                    |                       |
|      |                    |                       |
|      |                    |                       |
|      |                    |                       |
|      |                    |                       |
|      |                    |                       |
|      |                    |                       |
|      |                    |                       |
|      |                    |                       |
|      |                    |                       |
|      |                    |                       |
|      |                    |                       |
|      |                    |                       |
|      |                    |                       |
|      |                    |                       |
|      |                    |                       |
|      |                    |                       |
|      |                    |                       |
|      |                    |                       |
|      |                    |                       |
|      |                    |                       |
|      |                    |                       |
|      |                    |                       |
|      |                    |                       |
|      |                    |                       |
|      |                    |                       |
|      |                    |                       |
|      |                    |                       |
|      |                    |                       |
|      |                    |                       |
|      |                    |                       |
|      |                    |                       |
|      |                    |                       |
|      |                    |                       |

## Appointment Record
*Be sure to copy each form before you complete it.*
(Complete this log each time you schedule an appointment. Insert into your permanent file.)

| Provider | Date |
| --- | --- |
| | |
| | |
| | |
| | |
| | |
| | |
| | |
| | |
| | |
| | |
| | |
| | |
| | |
| | |
| | |
| | |
| | |
| | |
| | |
| | |
| | |
| | |
| | |
| | |
| | |
| | |
| | |
| | |
| | |
| | |
| | |
| | |
| | |
| | |
| | |
| | |
| | |
| | |
| | |
| | |
| | |
| | |
| | |
| | |
| | |

## Travel Log
*Be sure to copy each form before you complete it.*
(Complete this log after each trip you make. Insert into your permanent file.)

| Provider | Date | Miles |
|---|---|---|
|  |  |  |
|  |  |  |
|  |  |  |
|  |  |  |
|  |  |  |
|  |  |  |
|  |  |  |
|  |  |  |
|  |  |  |
|  |  |  |
|  |  |  |
|  |  |  |
|  |  |  |
|  |  |  |
|  |  |  |
|  |  |  |
|  |  |  |
|  |  |  |
|  |  |  |
|  |  |  |
|  |  |  |
|  |  |  |
|  |  |  |
|  |  |  |
|  |  |  |
|  |  |  |
|  |  |  |
|  |  |  |
|  |  |  |
|  |  |  |
|  |  |  |
|  |  |  |
|  |  |  |
|  |  |  |
|  |  |  |
|  |  |  |
|  |  |  |
|  |  |  |

## Reimbursement Record
*Be sure to copy each form before you complete it.*
(Complete this log each time you submit a bill or receive a check for reimbursement.
Insert into your permanent file.)

| Provider | Date Seen | Date Submitted | Date/Amount Reimbursed |
|---|---|---|---|
|  |  |  |  |
|  |  |  |  |
|  |  |  |  |
|  |  |  |  |
|  |  |  |  |
|  |  |  |  |
|  |  |  |  |
|  |  |  |  |
|  |  |  |  |
|  |  |  |  |
|  |  |  |  |
|  |  |  |  |
|  |  |  |  |
|  |  |  |  |
|  |  |  |  |
|  |  |  |  |
|  |  |  |  |
|  |  |  |  |
|  |  |  |  |
|  |  |  |  |
|  |  |  |  |
|  |  |  |  |
|  |  |  |  |
|  |  |  |  |
|  |  |  |  |
|  |  |  |  |
|  |  |  |  |
|  |  |  |  |
|  |  |  |  |
|  |  |  |  |
|  |  |  |  |
|  |  |  |  |
|  |  |  |  |
|  |  |  |  |
|  |  |  |  |
|  |  |  |  |
|  |  |  |  |
|  |  |  |  |
|  |  |  |  |
|  |  |  |  |
|  |  |  |  |
|  |  |  |  |
|  |  |  |  |

## Work Log
### *Be sure to copy each form before you complete it.*
(Complete this log each time you work so that you can have a log of the hours
for which you will be reimbursed. Insert into your permanent file.)

| Date | Hours Worked |
|------|--------------|
|      |              |
|      |              |
|      |              |
|      |              |
|      |              |
|      |              |
|      |              |
|      |              |
|      |              |
|      |              |
|      |              |
|      |              |
|      |              |
|      |              |
|      |              |
|      |              |
|      |              |
|      |              |
|      |              |
|      |              |
|      |              |
|      |              |
|      |              |
|      |              |
|      |              |
|      |              |
|      |              |
|      |              |
|      |              |
|      |              |
|      |              |
|      |              |
|      |              |
|      |              |
|      |              |
|      |              |
|      |              |
|      |              |
|      |              |
|      |              |

## *Appendix C – References and Resources*

| | |
|---|---|
| Agency for Healthcare Research and Quality www.ahcpr.gov | American Physical Therapy Association www.apta.org |
| American Academy of Allergy, Asthma & Immunology www.aaaai.org | Americans with Disabilities Act www.usdoj.gov/crt/ada/adahoml.htm |
| American Academy of Neurology www.aan.com | Association for Professionals in Infection Control and Epidemiology www.apic.org |
| American Academy of Orthopaedic Surgeons www.aaos.org | Association of Academic Physiatrists www.physiatry.org |
| American Academy of Pain Management www.aapainmanage.org | Association of National Health Occupational Physicians www.anhops.com |
| American Academy of Pain Medicine www.painmed.org | Association of Rehabilitation Nurses www.rehabnurse.org |
| American Association of Neurological Surgeons www.aans.org | The American Association for Hand Surgery www.handsurgery.org |
| American Association of Occupational Health Nursing www.aaohn.org | The American Health Quality Association www.ahqa.org |
| American Board of Medical Specialties www.agms.org | The American Occupational Therapy Association www.aota.org |
| American Cancer Society www.cancer.org | Centers for Disease Control and Prevention www.cdc.gov |
| American Chiropractic Association www.amerchiro.org | Centers for Medicare & Medicaid Services www.cms.hhs.gov |
| American College of Cardiology www.acc.org | Craig Hospital – Spinal Cord Injury and Traumatic Brain Injury Rehabilitation www.craighospital.org |
| American Diabetes Association www.diabetes.org | Department of Health and Human Services Centers for Disease Control www.cdc.gov |
| American Heart Association www.americanheart.org | Department of Veterans Affairs www.va.gov |
| American Lung Association www.lungusa.org | Emergency Medical Treatment and Labor Act Resource www.cms.hhs.gov/providers/emtala |
| American Massage Therapy Association www.amtamassage.org | ESA's *Office of Workers' Compensation Programs* www.dol.gov/dol/esa/public/owcp_org |
| American Medical Association www.ama-assn.org | The Health Insurance Portability & Accountability Act of 1996 www.cms.hhs.gov/hipaa |
| American Medical Association Doctor Finder dbapps.ama-assn.org/aps/amahg.htm | Infection Control Today www.infectioncontroltoday.com |
| American Neurological Association www.aneuroa.org | Infectious Diseases Society of America www.idsociety.org |
| American Nurses Association www.nursingworld.org | Johns Hopkins Hospital www.hopkinsmedicine.org |
| American Osteopathic Association www.osteopathic.org | Joint Commission on Accreditation of Healthcare Organizations www.jcaho.org |

| | |
|---|---|
| Mayo Clinic www.mayoclinic.org | Rehabilitation Act of 1973, Section 504 www.dol.gov.oasam/regs/statutes/sec504.htm |
| MedicineNet.com www.medicinenet.com | Social Security Administration www.ssa.gov |
| Medline Plus www.nlm.nih.gov/medlineplus | Social Security Disability Programs www.ssa.gov/disability |
| National Center for Infectious Disease www.cdc.gov/ncidod/diseases | The Family and Medical Leave Act of 1993 www.dol.gov/esa/regs/statutes/whd/fmla.htm |
| National Coordinating Council for Medication Error Reporting and Prevention www.nccmerp.org | The Merck Manuals www.merck.com |
| National Federation of the Blind www.nfb.org | U.S. Department of Health-National Institutes of Health www.nih.gov |
| National Institute of Allergy & Infectious Diseases www.niaid.nih.gov | U.S. Department of Justice-A Guide to Disability Rights Law www.usdoj.gov/crt/ada/cguide.htm |
| National Institutes of Health www.nih.gov | U.S. Department of Labor www.dol.gov |
| National Library of Medicine www.nlm.nig.gov/nlmhome.html | U.S. Department of Labor Bureau of Labor Statistics stats.bls/gov |
| National Mental Health Association www.nmha.org | U.S. Department of Labor Occupational Safety & Health Association www.osha.gov |
| National Practitioner Data Bank www.npdb-hipdb.com | U.S. Food and Drug Administration www.fda.gov |
| Occupational Outlook Handbook stats.bls.gov/oco/home.htm | |

## Alabama

Workers' Compensation Division—dir.alabama.gov/wc
Industrial Relations Building, 649 Monroe Street, Montgomery, Alabama 36131
(800) 528-5166, (334) 242-2868; Fax: (334) 353-8262 (Administrative/TPAs/Assessments/Self-Insurance), (334) 353-8228 (Examiners/Ombudsman), (334) 353-0840 (Claims), (334) 353-8490 (Compliance/Drug Free/Medical/Education); Fraud: (800) 923-2533; Ombudsman: (800) 528-5166, (334) 242-2868 (in Montgomery area)

## Alaska

Workers' Compensation Division—www.labor.state.ak.us/wc/wc.htm
Post Office Box 25512, Juneau, Alaska 99802-5512
(907) 465-2790; Fax: (907) 465-2797

## Arizona

Industrial Commission of Arizona—www.ica.state.az.us
800 West Washington, Phoenix, Arizona 85007
(602) 542-4411, Fax: (602) 542-7889; Ombudsman: (602) 542-4538, Fax: (602) 542-4350

## Arkansas

Workers' Compensation Commission—www.awcc.state.ar.us
Post Office Box 950, Little Rock, Arkansas 72203-0950
(800) 622-4472, (501) 682-3930; Fax: (501) 682-2777; Legal Advisor Direct: (800) 250-2511; TDD: (800) 285-1131 Arkansas Relay System TDD: (800) 285-1131

## California

Department of Industrial Relations—www.dir.ca.gov
Commission on Health and Safety and Workers' Compensation
(415) 557-1304, Fax: (415) 703-4234
Division of Workers' Compensation
Post Office Box 420603, San Francisco, California 94142

## Colorado

Division of Workers' Compensation—www.coworkforce.com/DWC
1515 Arapahoe Street, Tower 2, Suite 500, Denver, Colorado 80202-2117
(888) 390-7936, (800) 685-0891 (Spanish), (303) 575-8700, Fax: (303) 318-8710

## Connecticut

Workers' Compensation Commission—wcc.state.ct.us
Capitol Place, 21 Oak Street, Fourth Floor, Hartford, Connecticut 06106
(860) 493-1500, Fax: (860) 247-1361

## Delaware

Office of Workers' Compensation—www.delawareworks.com/industrialaffairs/services/workerscomp.shtml
State Office Building, Sixth Floor, 820 North French Street, Wilmington, Delaware 19801
(302) 761-8200, Fax: (302) 577-3750

### District of Columbia
Office of Workers' Compensation—www.does.dc.gov
Post Office Box 56098, Washington, District of Columbia 20002
(202) 671-1000, Fax: (202) 671-1929

### Florida
Division of Workers' Compensation—www.fldfs.com/WC
200 East Gaines Street, Tallahassee, Florida 32399-4220
(850) 921-6966; Fax: (850) 922-6779; Fraud: (800) 742-2214 (in Florida)
Department of Insurance, Bureau of Workers' Compensation Fraud: (850) 413-3116); Safety: (800) 367-4378 (in Florida), (850) 488-3044

### Georgia
Georgia State Board of Workers' Compensation—www.ganet.org/sbwc
270 Peachtree Street, NW, Atlanta, Georgia 30303-1299
(800) 533-0682, (404) 656-3875, Fax: (404) 656-7768, Enforcement Division: (404) 657-1391, Safety Library: (404) 656-9057

### Hawaii
Department of Labor & Industrial Relations—hawaii.gov/labor
Lorraine H. Akiba, Director, 830 Punchbowl Street, Honolulu, HI 96813
(808) 586-9151, Fax: (808) 586-9219

### Idaho
Industrial Commission—www2.state.id.us/iic
Post Office Box 83720, Boise, Idaho 83720-0041
(208)-334-6000, (208) 334-6000; Fax: (208) 334-2321; TDD: (800) 950-2110
State Insurance Fund—www.state.id.us/isif/index.htm
Post Office Box 83720, Boise, Idaho 83720-0044
(800) 334-2370, (208) 334-2370 (in the Boise area); Fax: (208) 334-2262 (Policyholder Services, Administration, Management Services, Legal), (208) 334-3253 (Claims), (208) 334-3254 (Underwriting); Fraud: (800) 448-ISIF (4743)

### Illinois
Industrial Commission—www.state.il.us/agency/iic
100 West Randolph Street, Suite 8-200, Chicago, Illinois 60601
(866) 352-3033, Fax: (312) 814-6523

### Indiana
Workers' Compensation Board of Indiana—www.in.gov/workcomp
Government Center South, 402 West Washington Street, Room W-196, Indianapolis, Indiana 46204
(317) 232-3809; Claims/Statistics: (317) 233-4930; Fax: (317) 233-5493; Insurance: (317) 233-3910; Ombudsman: (800) 824-COMP (2667), (317) 232-5922

### Iowa
Iowa Division of Workers' Compensation—www.state.ia.us/iwd/wc/index.html
1000 East Grand Avenue, Des Moines, Iowa 50319-0209
(800) JOB-IOWA (562-4692), (515) 281-5387; Fax: (515) 281-6501

## Kansas

Kansas Workers' Compensation—www.dol.ks.gov/wc/html/wc_ALL.html
800 SW Jackson, Suite 600, Topeka, Kansas 66612-1227
(785) 296-5000, (785) 296-3441; Fax: (785) 296-0839; Fraud: (800) 332-0353, (785) 296-6392;
Industrial Safety & Health: (800) 332-0353, (785) 296-4386;
Ombudsman: (800) 332-0353, (785) 296-2996

## Kentucky

Office of Workers' Claims—labor.ky.gov/dwc
657 Chamberlin Avenue, Frankfort, Kentucky 40601
(502) 564-5550 (Administrative Services, Open Records); Fax: (502) 564-8250 (Administrative
Services), (502) 564-9533 (Ombudsman), (502) 564-5732 (Open Records), (502) 564-0916 (Security and
Compliance); Ombudsman: (800) 554-8601 (Frankfort), (800) 554-8603 (Paducah), (800) 554-8602
(Pikeville); Security and Compliance: (502) 564-5550

## Louisiana

Office of Workers' Compensation Administration—www.ldol.state.la.us/bus_owca.asp
Post Office Box 94040, Baton Rouge, Louisiana 70804-9040
(225) 342-7555, Fax: (225) 342-5665, Fraud: (800) 201-3362, Safety: (800) 201-2497

## Maine

Workers' Compensation Board—www.state.me.us/wcb
27 State House Station, Augusta, Maine 04333-0027
(207) 287-3751; Fax: (207) 287-7198

## Maryland

Maryland Workers' Compensation Commission—www.wcc.state.md.us
10 East Baltimore Street, Baltimore, Maryland 21202
(800) 492-0479, (410) 864-5100; Fax: (410) 333-8122

## Massachusetts

Department of Industrial Accidents—www.state.ma.us/dia
600 Washington Street, 7th Floor, Boston, Massachusetts 02111
(800) 323-3249, (617) 727-4900; Fax: (617) 727-6477; TTY: (800) 224-6196
Massachusetts Workers' Compensation Advisory Council—www.state.ma.us/wcac/wcac.html
(617) 727-4900 x378, Fax: (617) 727-7122

## Michigan

Bureau of Workers' & Unemployment Compensation—www.michigan.gov/wca
Post Office Box 30016, Lansing, Michigan 48909
(888) 396-5041, (313) 456-2400, Fax: (313) 456-2424

## Minnesota

Workers' Compensation Division—www.doli.state.mn.us/workcomp.html
443 Lafayette Road North, St. Paul, Minnesota 55155
(800) DIAL-DLI (342-5354) in Greater Minnesota, (800) 342-5354 or (651) 284-5005 in the St. Paul
area, (800) 365-4584 or (218) 723-4670 in the Duluth area; Fax: (651) 282-5405; Fraud: (888) 372-8366,
(651) 297-5797, TDD: (651) 297-4198

## Mississippi

Mississippi Workers' Compensation Commission—www.mwcc.state.ms.us
Post Office Box 5300, Jackson, Mississippi 39296-5300
(601) 987-4200, Fraud: (601) 359-4250

## Missouri

Division of Workers' Compensation—www.dolir.state.mo.us/wc/index.htm
Post Office Box 58, Jefferson City, Missouri 65102-0058
(573) 751-4231, Fax: (573) 751-2012, Employee Hotline: (800) 775-2667, Employer Hotline: (888) 837-6069, Fraud and Noncompliance: (800)-592-6003, (573)-526-6630,
Workers' Safety Program: (573) 526-3504

## Montana

Montana State Fund—www.montanastatefund.com
Post Office Box 4759, Helena, Montana 59604-4759
(406) 444-6500, Claim Reporting/Customer Service: (800) 332-6102, Fraud Reporting: (888) 682-7463

## Nebraska

Workers' Compensation Court—www.nol.org/home/WC
State House, 13th Floor, Post Office Box 98908, Lincoln, Nebraska 68509-8908
(800) 599-5155 (in Nebraska only), (402) 471-6468 (Lincoln and out of state), Fax: (402) 471-2700

## Nevada

Division of Industrial Relations—dirweb.state.nv.us
400 West King Street, Suite 400, Carson City, Nevada 89703
(775) 684-7260, Fax: (775) 687-6305

## New Hampshire

Workers' Compensation Division—www.state.nh.us/dol/dol-wc/index.html
95 Pleasant Street, Concord, New Hampshire 03301
Claims: (603) 271-3174, Coverage: (603) 271-2042, Self-Insurance: (603) 271-6172,
Vocational Rehabilitation: (603) 271-3328

## New Jersey

Division of Workers' Compensation—www.nj.gov/labor/wc/wcindex.html
Post Office Box 381, Trenton, New Jersey 08625-0381
(609) 292-2515, Fax: (609) 984-2515

## New Mexico

Workers' Compensation Administration—www.state.nm.us/wca
Post Office Box 27198, Albuquerque, New Mexico 87125-7198
(800) 255-7965, (505) 841-6000, Fax: (505) 841-6009,
Help Line/Hot Line: (866) WORKOMP (967-5667)

## New York

New York State Workers' Compensation Board—www.wcb.state.ny.us
100 Broadway-Menands, Albany, New York 12241
(518) 474-6670, Fax: (518) 473-1415

## North Carolina
North Carolina Industrial Commission—www.comp.state.nc.us
4319 Mail Service Center, Raleigh, North Carolina 27699-4319
(919) 807-2500, Fax: (919) 715-0282
Fraud Investigations Section: (888) 891-4895—www.comp.state.nc.us/ncic/pages/fraud.htm
Ombudsman Section: (800) 688-8349—www.comp.state.nc.us/ncic/pages/ombudsmn.htm
Safety Education Section: (919) 807-2603—www.comp.state.nc.us/ncic/pages/safety.htm

## North Dakota
Workforce Safety & Insurance—www.WorkforceSafety.com
1600 East Century Avenue, Suite One, Bismarck, North Dakota 58506-5585
(800) 777-5033, (701) 328-3800; Fax: (701) 328-3820; Fraud: (800) 243-3331;
Safety and Loss Prevention: (701) 328-3886; TDD: (701) 328-3786

## Ohio
Ohio Bureau of Workers' Compensation—www.ohiobwc.com
30 West Spring Street, Columbus, Ohio 43215-2256
Industrial Commission of Ohio—www.ohioic.com/index.jsp
(800) 521-2691, (614) 466-6136, Fax: (614) 752-8304

## Oklahoma
Workers' Enforcement Compensation Division—www.okdol.state.ok.us/workcomp/index.htm
Department of Labor—www.okdol.state.ok.us
4001 North Lincoln Boulevard, Oklahoma City, Oklahoma 73105-5212
(888) 269-5353, (405) 528-1500 Fax: (405) 528-5751

## Oregon
Workers' Compensation Division —www.cbs.state.or.us/wcd
350 Winter Street NE, Room 27, Salem, Oregon 97301-3879
(800) 452-0288 (Workers' Compensation Infoline); (503) 947-7810, Fax: (503) 947-7514; TTY: (503) 947-7993; Fraud Hotline: (800) 422-8778 (in Oregon); Small Business Ombudsman: (503) 378-4209, Fax: (503) 373-7639; Ombudsman for Injured Workers: (800) 927-1271, (503) 378-3351
Workers' Compensation Board—www.cbs.state.or.us/wcb
2601 25th Street SE, Suite 150, Salem, Oregon 97302-1282
(503) 378-3308

## Pennsylvania
Bureau of Workers' Compensation—www.dli.state.pa.us
1171 South Cameron Street, Room 324, Harrisburg, Pennsylvania 17104-2501
(800) 482-2383 (inside Pennsylvania), (717) 772-4447 (local/out of state), TTY: (800) 362-4228

## Rhode Island
State of Rhode Island—www.state.ri.us
Workers' Compensation Court, One Dorrance Plaza, Providence, Rhode Island 02903
(401) 277-3097, Fax: (401) 421-3123

## South Carolina
Workers' Compensation Commission—www.wcc.state.sc.us
Post Office Box 1715, Columbia, South Carolina 29202-1715
(803) 737-5700, Fax: (803) 737-5768

## South Dakota
Division of Labor and Management—www.state.sd.us/dol/dlm/dlm-home.htm
Kneip Building, Third Floor, 700 Governors Drive, Pierre, South Dakota 57501-2291
(605) 773-3681, Fax: (605) 773-4211

## Tennessee
Workers' Compensation Division—www.state.tn.us/labor-wfd/wcomp.html
710 James Robertson Parkway, Gateway Plaza, Second Floor, Nashville, Tennessee 37243-0665
(800) 332-2667 (within Tennessee), (615) 532-4812, Fax: (615) 532-1468

## Texas
Texas Workers' Compensation Commission—www.twcc.state.tx.us
7551 Metro Center Drive, Suite 100, Austin, Texas 78744-1609
(512) 804-4000, Commissioners: (512) 804-4435 fax: (512) 804-4431, Customer Relations/Services:
(512) 804-4100 or 804-4636, Fax: (512) 804-4001, Fraud Hotline: (512) 804-4703, Injured Worker
Hotline/Ombudsman: (800) 252-7031, Safety Violations Hotline: (800) 452-9595

## Utah
Workers' Compensation Fund of Utah—www.wcf-utah.com
Salt Lake City Office, 392 East 6400 South, Murray, Utah 84107
(800) 446-2667

## Vermont
Workers' Compensation Division—www.state.vt.us/labind/wcindex.htm
National Life Building, Drawer 20, Montpelier, Vermont 05620-3401
(802) 828-2286, Fax: (802) 828-2195

## Virginia
Virginia Workers' Compensation Commission—www.vwc.state.va.us
1000 DMV Drive, Richmond, Virginia 23220
(877) 664-2566, Fax: (804) 367-9740, TDD: (804) 367-8600

## Washington
Workers' Compensation Information—www.lni.wa.gov/ClaimsInsurance
Department of Labor and Industries—www.lni.wa.gov
Labor and Industries Building, Post Office Box 44001, Olympia, Washington 98504-4001
(800) 547-8367, (360) 902-4213, Fax: (360) 902-4202

## West Virginia
Workers' Compensation Commission—www.wvwcc.org
Post Office Box 3824, Charleston, West Virginia 25338-3824
(888) 498-2667, (304) 926-5060, Fax: (304) 926-5372, Fraud: (800) 779-6853

## Wisconsin

Workers' Compensation Division—www.dwd.state.wi.us/wc/default.htm
Post Office Box 7901, Madison, Wisconsin 53707-7901
(608) 266-1340; Fax: (608) 267-0394; Fraud (608) 261-8486

## Wyoming

Workers' Safety and Compensation Division—wydoe.state.wy.us
Cheyenne Business Center, 1510 East Pershing Boulevard, Cheyenne, Wyoming 82002
(307) 777-5476, Fax: (307) 777-5524
To Report an Injury: (800) 870-8883 or (307) 777-7441, Fax: (307) 777-6552.
To Report Fraud: (888) 996-9226 or (307) 777-6552, Fax: (307) 777-3581.

## Navajo Nation

Navajo Nation—www.navajo.org
Workers' Compensation Program, Post Office Box 2489, Window Rock, Arizona 86515
(928) 871-6389, Fax: (928) 871-6087

## Puerto Rico

Puerto Rico—www.gobierno.pr
Industrial Commissioner's Office, G.P.O. Box 364466, San Juan, Puerto Rico 00936
(787) 783-3808, Fax: (787) 783-5610

## About the Author

Deborah Ribis has been a Registered Nurse for 23 years. Her vast experience has included working in trauma, intensive care, utilization management, medical care evaluation, and medical case management.

She has an intimate working knowledge of the workers' compensation, third party liability, managed care, and indemnity health care systems.

In her role as a Nationally Certified Nurse Life Care Planner, Deborah assessed the injured or ill individual as a whole; interpreted information received from the multi-disciplinary healthcare team, legal team, case management, and insurance carrier; and completed a Life Care Plan, used to identify and project lifetime medical, vocational, and personal care needs and costs for the injured or ill individual.

Deborah has also provided behind-the-scenes medical-legal consultation services for the insurance and legal industry with regard to issues of malpractice or liability.

## About the Editor

Brette McWhorter Sember is a retired attorney and mediator who is now the Senior Editor at Women in Print. Sember has authored over 20 books, and also teaches writing courses in addition to freelance writing and editing. Her web site is www.BretteSember.com.

## About the Copy Editor

Miriam S. Powell has pursued multiple career paths—from actress to software engineer to marketing drone—and has finally settled in as a freelance writer and editor. She now happily works on a variety of projects from her home in New England. Her web site is www.MiriamSPowell.com.

## About the Cover Designer

Mark A. Gitto provides graphic design services including logo creation, book design, business cards and web site design. You can reach him through us at Women In Print ® via email WomenInPrint@Surfglobal.net.

## Order Form

| Quantity | Title | Price | Total |
|---|---|---|---|
| | *Get Back On Your Feet!*<br>*What Every Injured and Ill Person Needs to Know*<br>ISBN: 0-974610901-0-7 *Deborah L. Ribis, RN, CNLCP* | $34.95 | |
| | Shipping Charges (see below) | | |
| | | Total | |

*Vermont residents add 7% sales tax.*

### Shipping Charges
UPS Ground, Federal Express Ground & Priority Mail

| First Book | $4.50 |
|---|---|
| Each Additional Book | Add $1.50 |

| Name | |
|---|---|
| Address | |
| City, State, Zip | |
| Telephone | |
| Email | |

Email confirmation of your order will be transmitted to the address provided.
This information will not be shared with any other parties.

Please mail completed order form and payment to us at:
### Women In Print®
PO Box 1527
Williston, VT 05495
Phone: 802-288-8040  Fax: 802-288-8041

We gladly accept credit cards through our web site www.WomenInPrint.com.